A BEGINNER'S GUIDE TO essential oils

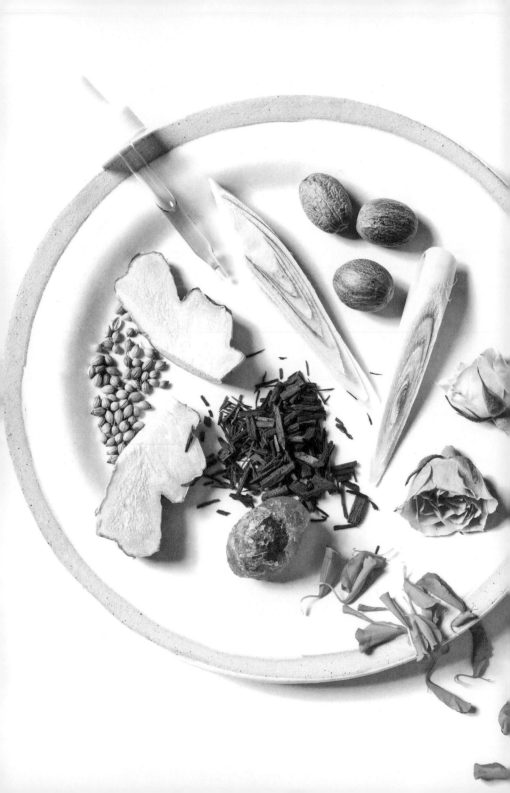

A BEGINNER'S GUIDE TO

essential oils

65+ ESSENTIAL OILS FOR
A HEALTHY MIND AND BODY

LISA BUTTERWORTH

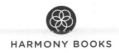

HARMONY BOOKS

CONTENTS

INTRODUCTION

Plants are magic. They're the unsung heroes of our life here on earth, cleaning our air, fortifying our soil, and, when properly used, healing our ailments. Essential oils offer us direct access to the curative power of plants, by distilling them to their essences and making their myriad benefits readily available, accessible, and, for the most part, affordable. They give us the ability to take our health into our own hands, and give us natural, easy ways to address a wide range of issues from the mental and emotional to the physical.

Natural plant remedies have been employed by humans for millennia, used for both preventative and reactive care. Today, even with all the wonders and benefits of modern medicine, essential oils are a marvelous way to tap into the natural world and help cultivate the knowledge and intuition necessary to enable us to tune in to ourselves, and take care of minds, bodies, and spirits.

If you are curious about essential oils, the following pages offer a general, easy-to-understand overview along with brief synopses of seventy specific oils: a perfect introduction to a time-tested way of healing.

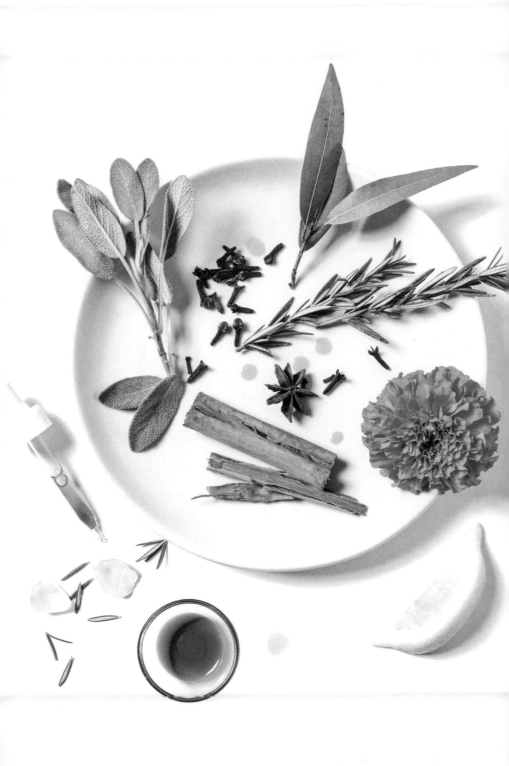

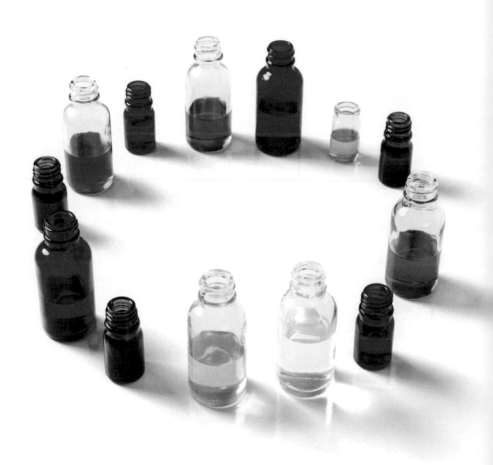

HOW TO USE ESSENTIAL OILS

Essential oils aren't actually oils. They are highly potent essences or concentrated compounds of the plant, tree, or flower they are made from. There are two main ways to benefit from essential oils: aromatically, by simply inhaling the oil, and topically, absorbing the oil through your skin. Each technique inspires a number of different methods for taking advantage of these essences. Twelve examples are listed below.

BATH
Baths are a wonderful self-care practice in and of themselves. Adding essential oils simply increases their healing potential. Essential oils can either be added directly to the bathwater or be mixed with carrier oil before being added. The warm water will help your skin absorb the essential oils in the bath, and you'll reap the aromatherapy benefits as well. Just be careful getting in and out of the tub—adding oil can make it slippery!

COMPRESS
Infusing a hot or cold compress—made using a folded facecloth and water—with an essential oil is a gentle way to reap an oil's benefits. Using a compress is a great method for treating joint pain, swelling, or cramps.

DIFFUSION
Diffusion is one of the easiest ways to enjoy an essential oil. Simply procure a diffuser—there are many kinds, so choose the one that suits you best— and use it in any (or every!) room of your home. You can foster a variety of particular environments with the scent alone, from calm and relaxed to cheery and stimulating. Oils can also freshen the air and fight the spread of airborne bacteria and viruses.

DIRECT APPLICATION
Applying an essential oil directly to the skin is a versatile way to treat a number of ailments. Essential oils can be applied undiluated or mixed in a salve, spray, or with carrier oil to treat insect bites, minor cuts and burns, and a variety of skin irritations. Just be sure to do a patch test (see page 15) to prevent any unwanted reaction.

DIRECT INHALATION
For aromatherapy on the go, it doesn't get easier than direct inhalation. To enjoy the oil's benefits, simply rub a drop between your palms, place them over your nose, and inhale, allowing the molecules instant access to your limbic system. You can also inhale directly from the bottle. Be sure to take several slow, deep breaths with either method.

FRAGRANCE
Many essential oils are used in commercial fragrances, and in the world of perfume their scent puts them in one of three categories: base note, middle note, or top note. As you become more familiar with essential oils, you can create a complex blend that synthesizes a scent just for you, but with several of the most delicious-smelling oils, you can also simply apply them directly for a lovely therapeutic aroma.

HOW TO USE ESSENTIAL OILS (CONTINUED)

HOME

Using essential oils in the home is a wonderful way to green your cleaning products. So many oils have antibacterial and antimicrobial properties, making them excellent agents for disinfecting everything from worktops in the kitchen to tiles in the bathroom. They also make excellent air fresheners, and you can reap their aromatherapy effects whether you're scrubbing dishes or wiping down mirrors. Oils can even have the power to turn chores into a mood-boosting experience.

INDIRECT INHALATION

Direct inhalation of an essential oil might be the quickest, most effective way to experience its benefits, but indirect inhalation is a great method, too. As mentioned earlier, a diffuser can be used for indirect inhalation, but there are other ways as well, including aromatic spritzers and simply putting a couple of drops on your pillowcase at night. Any topical method of application offers indirect inhalation benefits as well.

MASSAGE

Much like taking a bath, a massage is a powerful form of self-care, whether you engage in self-massage or receive it from another person. It's a way to wind down, soothe muscles, relax the mind and rejuvenate the spirit. Incorporating essential oils into this practice deepens its curative value. A general massage can restore or invigorate the body, while a targeted massage can alleviate pain or soreness. Using a carrier oil with an added essential oil tailored to your intention will not only soften and nourish your skin, it will also enhance the mental and physiological benefits.

SHOWER

For many of us, showering is something we do every day—an essential part of our personal grooming routine. Adding essential oils can take showering from a normal, mundane experience to one that has incredibly positive effects on your mood and well-being. Choose an oil depending on your need and enjoy its fragrance while also reaping its aromatherapy benefits.

SKIN, HAIR & MOUTH CARE

So many oils have positive effects on the skin and hair, from treating blemishes and softening fine lines to moisturizing hair and soothing an itchy scalp. And there are a number of ways to work essential oils into your skincare and beauty routine, giving you a boost inside and out. Some essential oils are also great for boosting the health of your mouth, mitigating bad breath, or treating ulcers.

STEAM INHALATION

When you're feeling under the weather, a steam inhalation of essential oils is a way to treat cold and flu symptoms, such as clogged sinuses, chest congestion, or a sore throat. Adding an essential oil to a hot bowl of water and breathing deeply as it steams will deliver the oil molecules into your nose and lungs, loosening mucus and soothing inflammation.

PAY ATTENTION TO QUALITY

The quality of essential oils can vary between brands, even if the label says each bottle holds the same oil. Be sure to procure your oils from a trusted source. Often, you get what you pay for. When you purchase an essential oil, make sure that the oil is the only ingredient in the bottle, and the bottle should be a dark blue or amber color to maintain the oil's integrity. Buy organic when possible, which will ensure that the matter used to make your essential oil was chemical and pesticide free, which in turn has a less negative effect on the environment as well.

SEVERAL THINGS TO KEEP IN MIND:

- Essential oils are highly concentrated and because of this, tiny doses can have big effects. If you're working with a new-to-you essential oil, start by using a small amount. You can always increase the amount of oil if you feel it's necessary.

- The relationship you cultivate with your oils is also important. Creating rituals around your self-care practice or being mindful as you put your oils to use can make them even more potent.

- Consider offering gratitude to the plant whose oil you're working with. Essential oils are the bridge that can help lead us to a synergistic relationship with the plant world. The oil you're about to use is a gift from the earth; treating it as such will only enhance the healing process.

CARRIER OILS

Because essential oils are highly concentrated, they should almost always be diluted when using them topically. Carrier oils are a great way to do this. Simply add the essential oil(s) you're using to a carrier oil before applying it to your skin. Different carrier oils have different benefits; choose the one that best fits your intended effect. Here are ten widely used carrier oils, along with their different benefits.

Apricot kernel oil: This oil is cold pressed from the cores of apricot stones. Similar in makeup to sweet almond oil, it is also light, versatile, and easily absorbed, but even more gentle for those with sensitive skin.

Argan oil: Rich but light, argan oil is most often used for hair and skincare because of its easy absorption. Cold pressed from the kernels of *Argania spinosa*, the Moroccan argan tree.

Avocado oil: This oil is from the flesh of the fruit. It is rich and highly hydrating, with vitamins A and E, but very thick. Look for cold-pressed avocado oil to avoid overprocessing.

Coconut oil: A great general moisturizer, and though it solidifies at room temperature, this oil melts quickly, or upon touch. If you have oily or acne-prone skin, it might be too heavy for use in facial blends. It has a faint aroma of coconut that does not overpower.

Grapeseed oil: This light, nourishing oil comes from the seeds of grapes, and hydrates the skin without leaving it greasy. Look for cold-pressed oil to avoid excess chemicals.

Jojoba oil: This oil comes from the seed of the *Simmondsia chinensis*, a desert shrub. It is thick and waxy and resembles our natural sebum more than any other carrier oil, making it great for skincare purposes.

Olive oil: Expressed from olives, this oil, which is a culinary staple, can also be used as a carrier, though it has an oily feel and can sometimes have an overpowering aroma. Look for cold-pressed oil to avoid overprocessing.

Rosehip oil: A gentle, hydrating oil, this is cold pressed from the seeds of the rosehip fruit, and because it is nongreasy, it is often used for skincare purposes. Store in the fridge.

Sunflower oil: A versatile oil, this is one of the more affordable carrier oils. It is light, easily absorbed, and very nourishing for the skin because it is rich in fatty acids as well as vitamins A, D, and E.

Sweet almond oil: This oil offers another affordable carrier oil option. The same almonds we snack on are the ones that are pressed to create this light, subtle oil, which contains lots of fatty acids and is rich in vitamin E, making it great for skin.

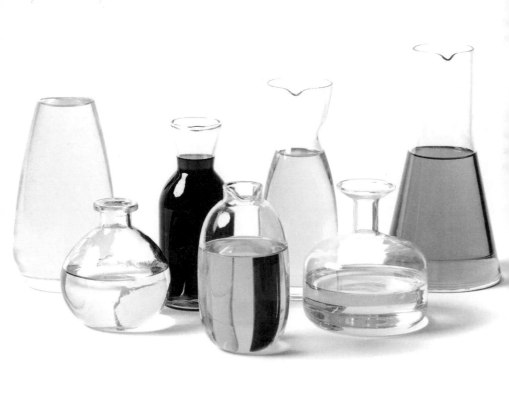

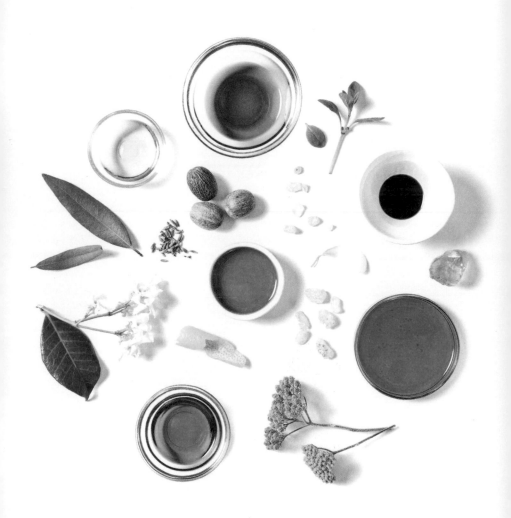

USING ESSENTIAL OILS SAFELY

Although it's been mentioned previously, it bears repeating: Essential oils are highly concentrated compounds, and while many are entirely safe, there are some precautions you should take.

 Sensitive skin: Some oils may cause a reaction in users with sensitive skin, and any oil may cause skin irritation if an individual reacts to its particular makeup. To be safe, conduct a patch test before using it by diluting the essential oil in a carrier oil and applying it to a small patch of skin. Leave overnight and then check for a reaction.

 Pregnant & breastfeeding: Women in the first trimester of pregnancy should refrain from using essential oils. After the first trimester and while breastfeeding, essential oils should be used with caution, and limited to the oils that are deemed safe for pregnancy.

 Children & elderly: Though some oils are safe for children, a very low dosage should be used, and each oil should be researched before put into use. The dosage of essential oils used should be minimized for the elderly as well, as they may be more sensitive to the oils' potency.

 Ingestion: Though it is a common practice to ingest oils, because of their high concentration and volatility, it is not a method suggested here. Consult an aromatherapist or medical practitioner first.

 Photosensitivity: Some oils cause a reaction to sunlight when applied to the skin, an effect known as photosensitivity. Refrain from using photosensitive oils on skin that will be exposed to sunlight within twelve to twenty-four hours.

 Medical conditions & pharmaceutical use: Some oils may have contraindications for users who have existing medical conditions (e.g., cancer, epilepsy, high blood pressure) or are taking medications. Research each oil before use, and consult a medical practitioner if you have any questions or concerns.

 Storage: Oils and blends should be kept in amber or dark blue glass bottles, with secure lids. Store your oils in a cool, dark place. Keep out of the reach of children.

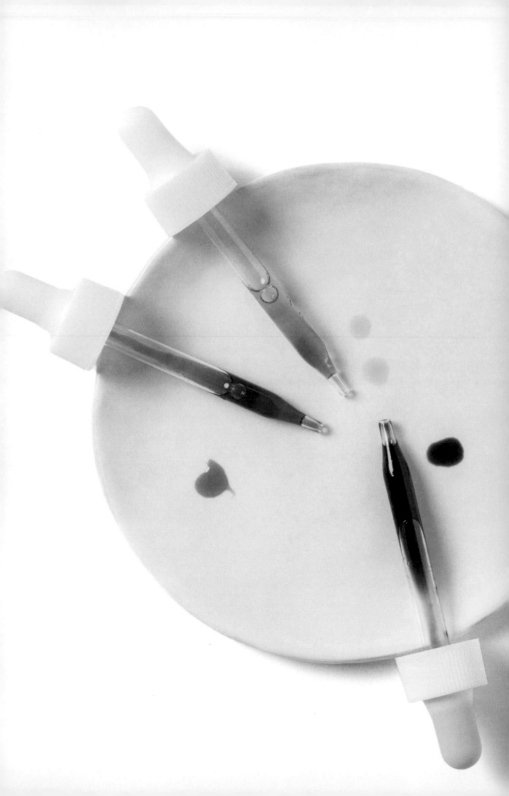

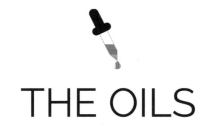

THE OILS

A guide to working with essential oils

BLUE CHAMOMILE

Matricaria recutita

 Use it for: Soothing itching and irritation, easing inflammation, increasing relaxation, supporting sleep, nourishing skin.

 Blend it with: Lavender and peppermint to help relieve insect bites; cypress has similar anti-inflammatory properties; eucalyptus deepens blue chamomile's relaxing properties; ylang-ylang also soothes skin.

What is it?: The small, daisy-like flowers of *Matricaria recutita* are steam distilled to create blue chamomile oil, also known as German chamomile. The essential oil, which is similar in makeup to Roman chamomile, is blue in color and has a sweet, earthy scent; it's widely used for its calming properties that benefit both the mind and the body.

Be safe: Blue chamomile may cause drowsiness and may irritate sensitive skin, so do a patch test before using.

TRY IT OUT:

 Bath: For a skin-soothing and relaxing bath, add 4 drops of blue chamomile and 2 drops of ylang-ylang to a tablespoon of a carrier oil and add to a warm bath.

 Indirect inhalation: Set the stage for a good night's sleep by adding a couple of drops of blue chamomile to your pillowcase before going to bed.

 Direct application: To reduce the itch and swelling of insect bites or stings, mix 1 drop of blue chamomile and 1 drop of lavender with 1 drop of a carrier oil and use your finger to apply it directly to the bite or sting.

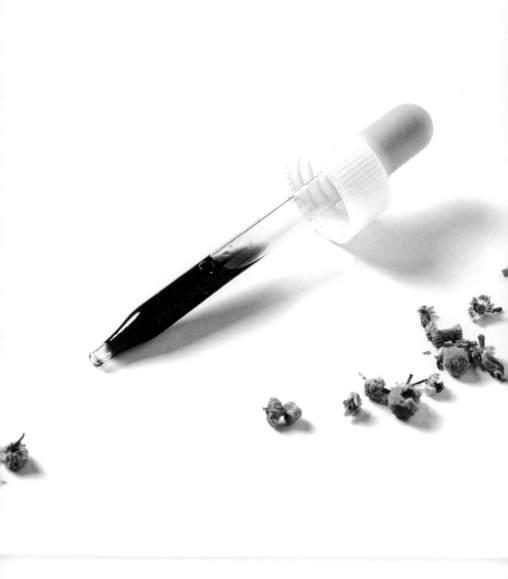

GERANIUM

Pelargonium graveolens

 Use it for: Nourishing skin, boosting hair health, repelling insects, calming anxiety, enhancing circulation.

 Blend it with: Citronella and lemongrass are also insect deterrents; tea tree can help problem skin; jasmine helps tone and balance skin; ylang-ylang enhances geranium's mood-lifting properties.

What is it?: The flowers and deep green leaves of *Pelargonium graveolens*, a shrub with pink or white blooms, are distilled to create geranium essential oil. This subtly rose-scented oil has wonderfully calming properties for the skin and the mind.

Be safe: Geranium may irritate sensitive skin, so do a patch test before using. Do not use geranium while pregnant. Geranium may cause drowsiness.

TRY IT OUT:

 Bath: For a calming, detoxifying bath, add 5 drops of geranium oil to a teaspoon of a carrier oil. Add blend to 3½ ounces (100g) of Epsom salt in a lidded jar and shake so the oil is evenly dispersed. Add the salt mixture to a warm bath.

 Hair care: Strengthen your hair and add some luster with this geranium hot oil treatment. Mix 1 ounce (30g) melted, warm coconut oil with 8 drops of geranium. Massage into dry or damp hair from scalp to ends, then cover with a warm towel for 20 minutes to an hour. Wash as usual.

 Skincare: For a soothing face mask that can treat blemishes and brighten skin, add 2 drops of geranium to 1 tablespoon (15g) raw honey and 2 teaspoons (10g) of aloe vera gel. Apply with fingertips to a clean, dry face. Leave on for 15 minutes, then remove with warm water.

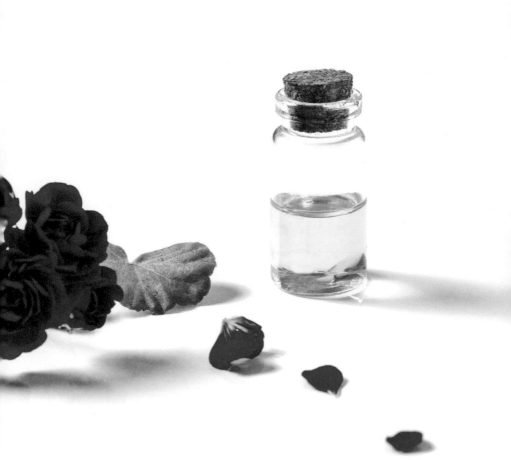

HELICHRYSUM

Helichrysum italicum

 Use it for: Reducing scarring, soothing skin inflammation, healing cuts and scrapes, boosting skin health, supporting difficult emotions.

 Blend it with: Tea tree boosts its acne-fighting properties; cypress and blue chamomile also help soothe inflammation; geranium adds skin-smoothing qualities; lavender increases helichrysum's antiseptic properties.

What is it?: *Helichrysum italicum* is a long-stemmed herb topped with clusters of small yellow flowers. The leaves and flowers of this plant, which is also known as immortelle, are steam distilled to create helichrysum essential oil. It has a sweet earthy scent and is best known for its many skin benefits.

Be safe: Do not use helichrysum while pregnant or breastfeeding.

TRY IT OUT:

 Skincare: To boost your skin's texture and reduce the appearance of fine lines or sunspots, add helichrysum to your beauty routine. Place a single-use amount of your nightly moisturizer in your palm and add 1 drop of helichrysum before applying to your face.

 Compress: Lessen the severity of a bruise by creating a cold compress. Mix 5 drops of helichrysum and 3 drops of geranium in a cup of cold water. Take a clean, folded facecloth and place it on top of the water, letting it soak up as much oil and water as possible. Wring out the water and place the compress on the bruise.

 Direct application: Helichrysum is known for its ability to heal skin. To reduce scarring, apply a couple of drops of helichrysum directly to a cut or scrape as it heals. Repeat twice daily. Helichrysum can also be applied to older scars, though its effect will be diminished.

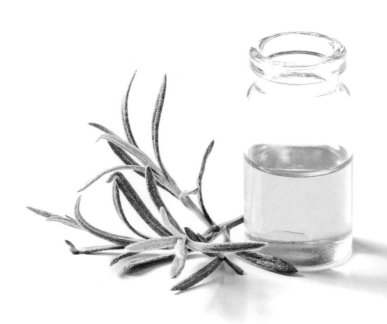

JASMINE

Jasminum officinale

 Use it for: Improving concentration, enhancing feelings of well-being, mitigating premenstrual syndrome (PMS), boosting skin health.

 Blend it with: Geranium is also good for balancing skin; rose is similarly emotionally soothing; clary sage and Roman chamomile help support menstrual-related symptoms; sandalwood adds an aromatic spice to jasmine's floral scent.

What is it?: The small, white fragrant flowers of *Jasminum officinale* are carbon dioxide or solvent extracted to create jasmine absolute. Because of the large amount of flowers it takes to create a small amount of absolute (about 1 million pounds of flowers to create 2½ pounds of absolute), jasmine is on the pricier side. Its warm floral scent is a perfumery mainstay, but jasmine has many emotionally therapeutic effects as well.

Be safe: Do not use jasmine while pregnant or breastfeeding.

TRY IT OUT:

 Diffusion: Diffuse jasmine in the home to create a supportive environment and sense of well-being.

 Fragrance: The light floral scent of jasmine is a natural perfume and can also boost optimism and confidence throughout the day; place 1 drop of jasmine on the inside of each wrist.

 Compress: To alleviate the discomfort of menstrual cramps, create a hot compress by mixing 6 drops of jasmine in 1 cup (250ml) hot water. Take a clean, folded facecloth and place it on top of the water, letting it soak up as much oil and water as possible. Wring out the water and place the compress on your abdomen.

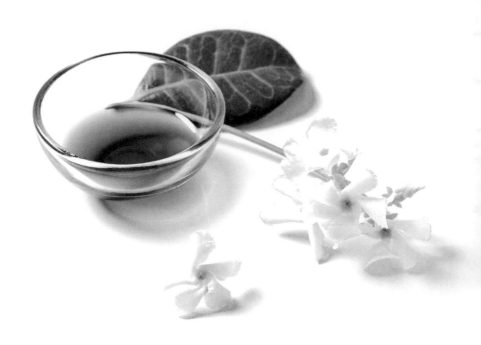

LAVANDIN

Lavandula x intermedia

 Use it for: Relieving anxiety, relaxing the mind, treating blemishes, soothing sore muscles, alleviating menstrual cramps.

 Blend it with: Tea tree and lemongrass are also good for treating problem skin; clary sage similarly soothes anxiety; juniper and sweet marjoram can also ease muscle pain.

What is it?: Lavandin is the result of cross-pollination between English lavender (*Lavandula angustifolia*) and Portuguese lavender (*Lavandula latifolia*); it's a tall-stemmed bush with deep purple flowering tops, which are steam distilled to create lavandin essential oil. The scent of this fragrance mainstay is less floral than lavender,and though it doesn't have lavender's versatility, it does have a number of therapeutic benefits.

Be safe: There are no known precautions associated with lavandin oil.

TRY IT OUT:

 Diffusion: For a calm environment that enhances concentration, diffuse lavandin and clary sage in the home.

 Skincare: To create an acne-fighting toner, mix 6 drops of lavandin, 2 drops of lavender, and 2 drops of tea tree in ¼ cup (50ml) of witch hazel in a small amber or dark blue bottle. Dab onto a cotton ball and wipe over your face after cleansing. Shake before each use.

 Compress: To create a compress that will help alleviate the pain of menstrual cramps while reducing stress, mix 4 drops of lavandin and 2 drops of juniper berry in 1 cup (250ml) hot water. Take a clean, folded facecloth and place it on top of the water, letting it soak up as much oil and water as possible. Wring out the water and place the compress on your abdomen.

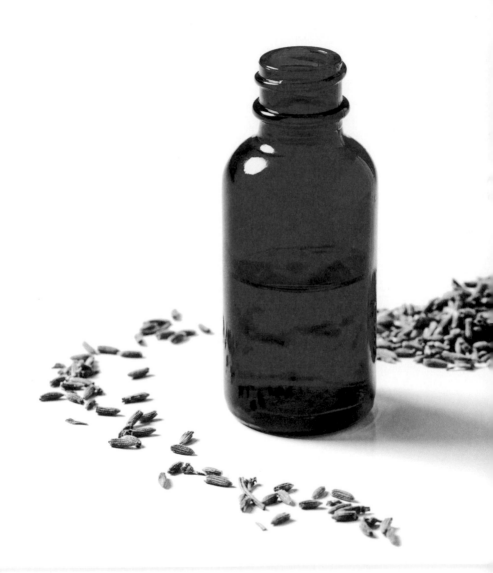

LAVENDER

Lavandula angustifolia

 Use it for: Treating insomnia, easing anxiety, alleviating headaches and migraines, promoting calm, soothing muscle tension.

 Blend it with: Blue chamomile and Roman chamomile are similarly soothing and relaxing; eucalyptus and tea tree share lavender's antiseptic qualities; the citrus scent of sweet orange pairs well with lavender's floral fragrance and adds a sense of well-being.

What is it?: Lavender oil is steam distilled from the flowering tops of *Lavandula angustifolia,* a tall-stemmed bush that blossoms with flowers in varying shades of purple.

Because of its versatility, lavender is indispensable when building an essential oil collection—it has as many physical benefits as it does mental and emotional.

Be safe: Lavender may cause drowsiness.

TRY IT OUT:

 Direct inhalation: To ease headache pain or stave off the oncoming effects of a migraine, rub 1 drop of lavender between your palms, place hands over your nose, and inhale deeply.

 Massage: Tend to muscle pain and tension by creating a massage oil. Add 15 drops of lavender to 2 tablespoons (30ml) of a carrier oil (scale up as needed). Blend and massage directly into skin.

 Indirect inhalation: To encourage a deep and restful sleep, add a couple of drops of lavender to your pillowcase before going to bed.

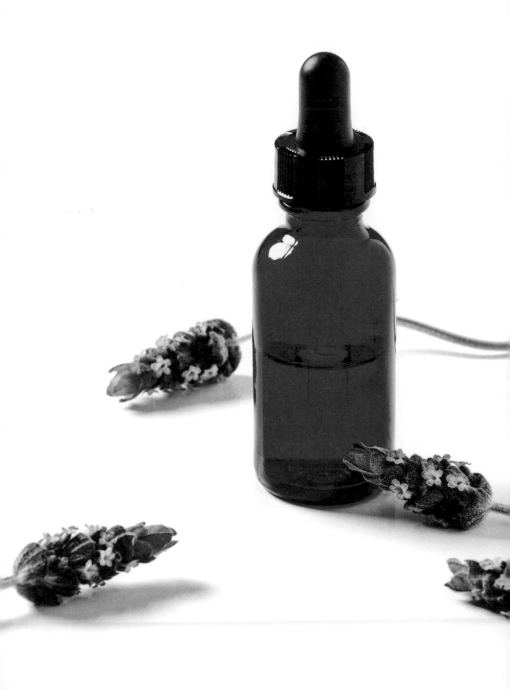

MANUKA

Leptospermum scoparium

 Use it for: Balancing skin, fighting bacteria, alleviating fungal infections, soothing nerves, relieving the itch and sting of insect bites.

 Blend it with: Palmarosa and geranium enhance manuka's skincare benefits; lavender and Roman chamomile amp up its relaxation properties; grapefruit adds emotional uplift.

What is it?: The leaves and twigs of *Leptospermum scoparium*, a flowering shrub native to New Zealand and Australia, are steam distilled to create manuka essential oil. Sweet, earthy, with a medicinal hint, manuka oil has similar analgesic, antiseptic, and anti-inflammatory properties to tea tree oil but is more suitable for those with sensitive skin.

Be safe: Do not use manuka internally.

TRY IT OUT:

 Home: For a purifying air freshener and aromatic spritz, add 12 drops of manuka and 6 drops of grapefruit to 2 tablespoons (30ml) water. Shake, spray, and inhale deeply.

 Skincare: To create a toner that helps balance skin and prevent acne, add 6 drops of manuka to 2 tablespoons (30ml) of witch hazel in a small amber or dark blue bottle. To use, shake to blend, dab onto a cotton ball, and wipe over your face after cleansing.

 Direct application: To take the itch and/or sting out of an insect bite, apply 1 drop of manuka directly to the bite.

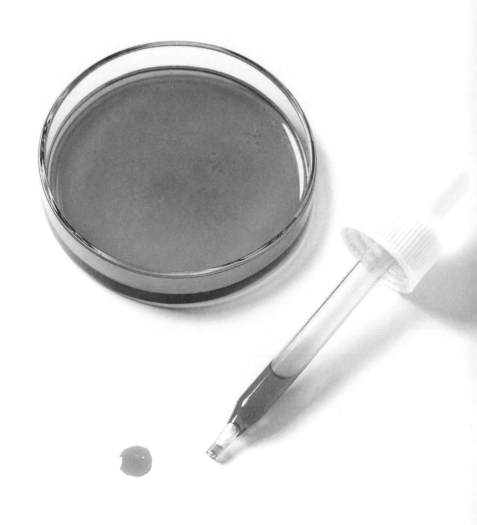

NEROLI

Citrus aurantium

 Use it for: Promoting sleep, easing anxiety, boosting skin health, lifting emotions, alleviating headaches.

 Blend it with: Petitgrain and Roman chamomile enhance neroli's relaxing properties; mandarin amps up its mood-boosting effect; geranium and jasmine similarly nourish skin.

What is it?: Because it takes an immense amount of flowers from *Citrus aurantium*, the bitter orange tree, to create 1 ounce neroli essential oil, this is one of the pricier oils available. (The more affordable petitgrain essential oil is distilled from the tree's leaves and twigs.) But you might decide that its bright floral scent alone is worth the cost. It's also a potent mood booster, sleep enhancer, and skincare beneficent.

Be safe: Neroli may cause drowsiness.

TRY IT OUT:

 Bath: For a relaxing bath that will prep you for a good night's sleep while also nourishing your skin, add 6 drops of neroli to a tablespoon of a carrier oil and add to a warm bath.

 Diffusion: For a pleasing fragrance that also creates a buoyant atmosphere, diffuse neroli in the home, especially in the evening to foster the transition from a busy, stressful day.

 Skincare: Freshen up your skin with a neroli facial mist: mix 2 tablespoons (30ml) water and 2 tablespoons (30ml) of witch hazel in a small amber or dark blue spray bottle. Add 7 drops of neroli and shake to blend before each use.

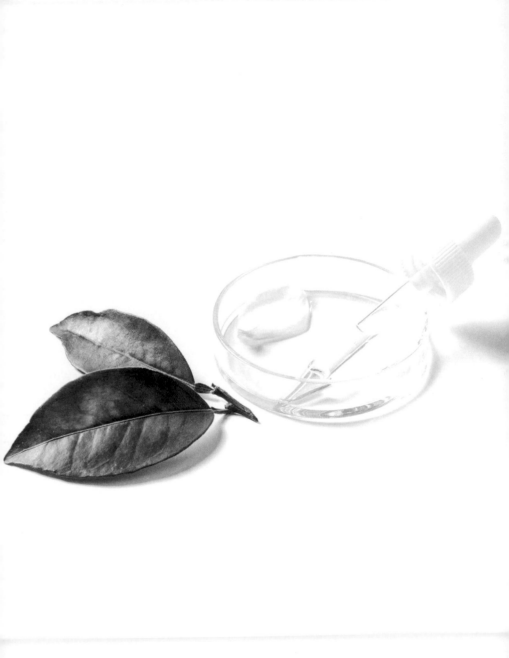

PALMAROSA

Cymbopogon martinii

 Use it for: Healing dry skin, uplifting emotions, enhancing sleep, promoting hair health, preventing infections.

 Blend it with: Lemongrass and rose are also beneficial for skin; patchouli is similarly moisturizing; lavender increases palmarosa's calming properties; myrrh is also helpful for treating cuts and scrapes.

What is it?: The leaves of *Cymbopogon martinii*—a long-leafed, flowering grass—are steam distilled to create palmarosa, a sweet, subtle oil with floral and citrus notes. It offers a reliable boost for both mental and skin health.

Be safe: Palmarosa may irritate sensitive skin, so do a patch test before using. Do not use palmarosa while pregnant.

TRY IT OUT:

 Bath: For a soothing bath that will usher in a good night's sleep, add 3 drops of palmarosa and 2 drops of lavender to a tablespoon of a carrier oil and add to a warm bath.

 Hair care: To reap palmarosa's hair health benefits, try a hot oil treatment. Mix 1 tablespoon melted coconut oil with 1 tablespoon jojoba oil in a small jar. Add 5 drops of palmarosa, 2 drops of Roman chamomile, and 1 drop of clary sage. Place the jar in a bowl of hot water until the oil is warm. Massage into dry or damp hair from scalp to ends, then cover hair with a warm towel for 20 minutes to an hour. Wash as usual.

 Skincare: To create a refreshing, moisturizing face mist, mix 2 tablespoons (30ml) water with 1 tablespoon (15g) of aloe vera juice in a small amber or dark blue spray bottle. Add 3 drops of palmarosa and 2 drops of rose. Mist over your face after cleansing or when you'd like to freshen up.

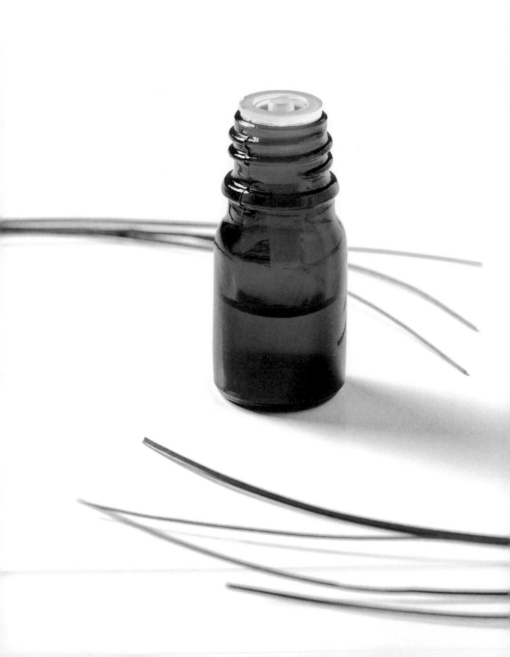

PETITGRAIN

Citrus aurantium

 Use it for: Abating insomnia, reducing anxiety, calming emotional flare-ups, soothing muscle spasms, treating acne, and boosting skin health.

 Blend it with: Lavender and ylang-ylang are also sleep aids; valerian has similarly potent relaxing properties; citrus scents, such as sweet orange and tangerine, complement petitgrain's floral aroma.

What is it?: The leaves and twigs of *Citrus aurantium*, also known as the bitter orange tree, are steam distilled to create petitgrain essential oil, which boasts an intoxicating scent featuring floral, citrus, and woody notes. (The tree's blossoms are distilled to create neroli essential oil.) In addition to its well-loved aroma, petitgrain has many emotionally therapeutic benefits and is often used in skincare as well.

Be safe: Petitgrain may cause drowsiness.

TRY IT OUT:

 Fragrance: Wear petitgrain as a fragrance by placing 1 drop of oil on the inside of each wrist, to take advantage of its woody, floral scent while reaping its de-stressing benefits.

 Shower: For a relaxing transition from day to night, enjoy an evening shower with all of petitgrain's calming benefits. After washing, with the hot water still running, apply 3 drops of petitgrain to a facecloth and rub it over your body, inhaling deeply as you do.

 Skincare: Treat problem skin by making a toner: in a small amber or dark blue bottle, add 4 drops of petitgrain and 2 drops of lavender to 2 tablespoons (30ml) of witch hazel. To use, shake to blend, dab onto a cotton ball, and wipe over your face after cleansing.

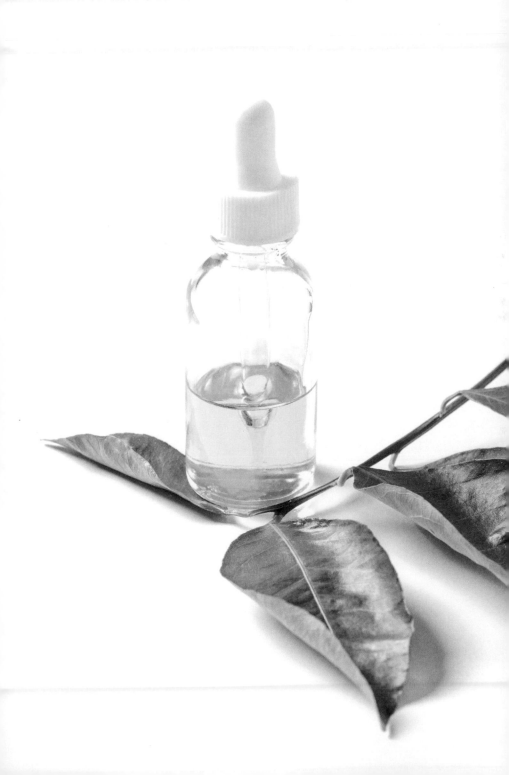

ROMAN CHAMOMILE

Anthemis nobilis

 Use it for: Calming the mind, promoting sleep, treating insect bites and stings, soothing skin, treating muscle spasms.

 Blend it with: Vetiver also promotes sleep; myrrh enhances Roman chamomile's soothing properties; cypress and lavender are also anti-inflammatory; peppermint boosts Roman chamomile's cooling effects.

What is it?: *Anthemis nobilis* is a small, leafy plant whose tiny white flowers are steam distilled to create Roman chamomile essential oil. This oil's sweet, floral, subtly fruity scent differentiates it from blue chamomile, and its similar properties—soothing skin and spirit—are just slightly stronger.

Be safe: Roman chamomile may cause drowsiness. Do not use while pregnant.

TRY IT OUT:

 Direct inhalation: For an immediate path into deep relaxation, rub 1 drop of Roman chamomile between your palms, place your hands over your nose, and inhale deeply.

 Massage: Ease your mind and muscles with this massage oil: Add 10 to 15 drops of Roman chamomile to 2 tablespoons (30ml) of a carrier oil. Blend and massage directly into skin.

 Direct application: To take the heat out of a sunburn and calm the inflamed skin, create a soothing spray. In a small amber or dark blue spray bottle, add 8 drops of Roman chamomile and 3 drops of peppermint to ¼ cup (50ml) of aloe vera juice. Shake to blend before using and spray onto the affected area.

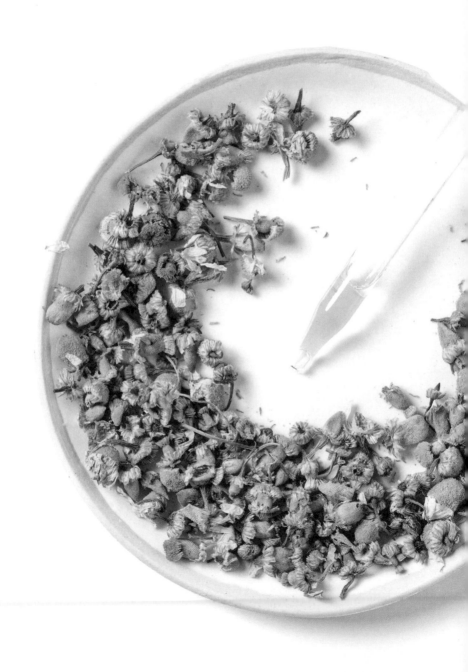

ROSE

Rosa damascena

 Use it for: De-stressing, alleviating depression, tempering emotions, rejuvenating skin, mitigating symptoms of PMS.

 Blend it with: Jasmine also helps balance emotions; geranium enhances skin health; blue chamomile and ylang-ylang give rose a relaxing boost; sandalwood gives rose's floral scent a rich, woody depth.

What is it?: Hundreds of thousands of petals from the fragrant flowers of the thorny *Rosa damascena* are solvent extracted to create just 1 ounce (30g) of rose absolute, making it one of the most valuable oils you can buy. Thankfully, a little goes a long way when it comes to this sweetly fragrant floral oil, which has many emotional benefits and is great for skincare, too.

Be safe: Do not use rose while pregnant.

TRY IT OUT:

 Bath: For a soothing bath that will also nourish the skin, add 5 drops of rose and 2 drops of geranium to a tablespoon of a carrier oil and add to a warm bath.

 Fragrance: Rose is a classic fragrance for good reason. Use this oil as a natural perfume, which can also provide comfort and emotional support throughout the day; place 1 drop of rose on the inside of each wrist.

 Skincare: To boost skin elasticity and radiance while adding a luxurious scent to your bedtime routine, add 1 drop of rose to a single-use amount of your nightly moisturizer before applying it to your face.

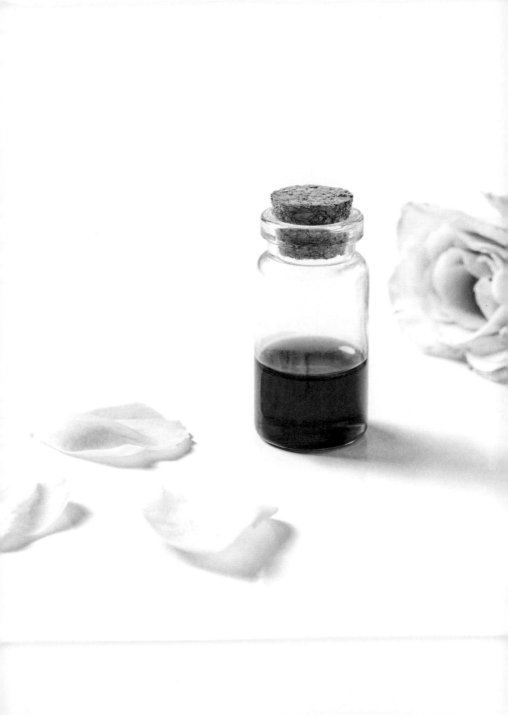

ROSE GERANIUM

Pelargonium roseum

 Use it for: Boosting skin health, balancing emotions, easing symptoms of PMS, promoting well-being, treating cuts and scrapes.

 Blend it with: Bergamot and lavender make rose geranium an emotionally supportive powerhouse; ylang-ylang is also a skin soother; neroli boosts its moisturizing properties; jasmine helps mitigate PMS, too.

What is it?: The leaves of *Pelargonium roseum*, an uncommon species of geranium with pink to white flowers, are steam distilled to create rose geranium essential oil. With a lovely floral scent that has herbaceous hints as well as citrus notes, this oil is wonderful for saving skin and sanity alike.

Be safe: Do not use rose geranium while pregnant.

TRY IT OUT:

 Bath: For a relaxing, uplifting soak for menstrual support, mix 2 drops of rose geranium, 2 drops of bergamot, and 1 drop of jasmine in a tablespoon of a carrier oil and add to a warm bath.

 Indirect inhalation: For a portable sense of calm and support, create this aromatic spritzer: add 12 drops of rose geranium, 10 drops of bergamot, and 8 drops of myrrh to a portable spray bottle. Fill the bottle with water. To use, spray in the air and walk through it, inhaling deeply.

 Direct application: To speed the healing of a cut, scrape, or other small wound, mix a couple of drops of rose geranium with a couple of drops of a carrier oil and apply to the affected area after cleansing.

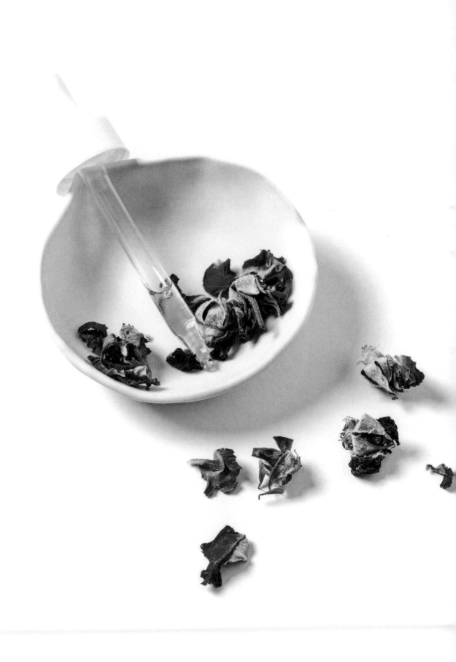

YLANG-YLANG

Cananga odorata

 Use it for: Increasing relaxation, decreasing blood pressure, easing depression, treating dry skin, and soothing skin irritation.

 Blend it with: Geranium and rose have similar skin-balancing qualities; tea tree shares ylang-ylang's antiseptic benefits; the citrus scent of sweet orange complements ylang-ylang's floral aroma; vetiver also lifts emotions.

What is it?: The vibrant yellow flowers of *Cananga odorata*, a tropical tree native to Southeast Asia, are steam distilled to create the sweetly floral, very fragrant ylang-ylang oil. It is often used in perfumes and is known for its skin and hair care benefits.

Be safe: Ylang-ylang may cause drowsiness. It may irritate sensitive skin, so do a patch test before using.

TRY IT OUT:

 Diffusion: Diffuse ylang-ylang in the home to create a calm environment.

 Fragrance: For a floral scent that can uplift your mood throughout the day, place 1 drop of ylang-ylang on the inside of each wrist.

 Skincare: To treat oily, combination, or acne-prone skin, place a single-use amount of your nightly moisturizer in your palm and add 1 drop of ylang-ylang before applying it to your face.

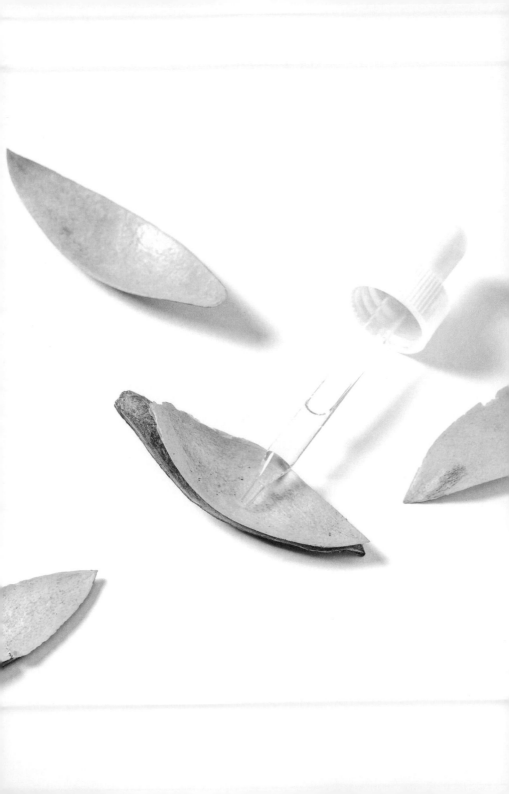

BASIL

Ocimum basilicum

 Use it for: Reenergizing, alleviating headaches, soothing insect bites, treating infections, boosting circulation.

 Blend it with: Lemon can also reduce headache pain; peppermint alleviates the itch of insect bites; citronella and rosemary have similar alertness-boosting properties; tea tree is also antiseptic.

What is it?: *Ocimum basilicum,* better known as the leafy, culinary mainstay herb basil, is harvested when flowering and the leaves are steam distilled to create basil essential oil. This sweet and spicy oil has a hint of licorice, and many stimulating benefits, in addition to being antiseptic and antibacterial.

Be safe: Do not use basil internally. Do not use basil while pregnant or breastfeeding. If you have epilepsy or are prone to seizures, refrain from use.

TRY IT OUT:

 Massage: For a warm, stimulating foot rub, try this massage oil: add 3 drops of basil and 2 drops of ginger to 1 tablespoon (15ml) of a carrier oil. Apply directly to sore feet to boost circulation and reenergize.

 Direct application: To treat a headache, mix 1 drop of basil with 1 drop of a carrier oil and use your finger to massage it into each temple, inhaling deeply as you do.

 Direct application: To alleviate the discomfort of insect bites, dilute a couple of drops of basil with a couple of drops of a carrier oil. Use your finger to dab directly onto a bite.

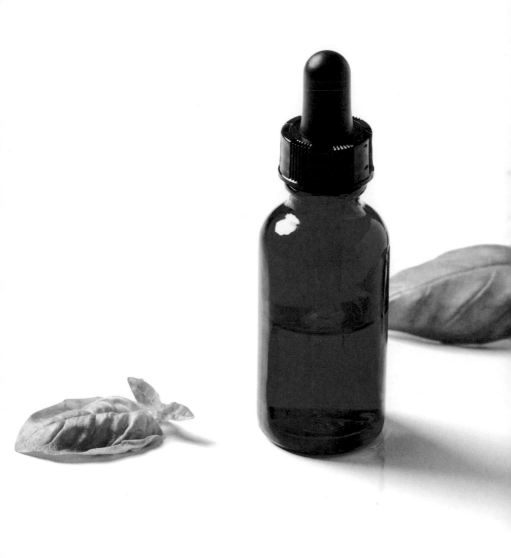

BAY LAUREL

Laurus nobilis

 Use it for: Soothing sore muscles, boosting confidence, reenergizing, supporting the lymphatic system, alleviating dry scalp and hair.

 Blend it with: Cardamom and clary sage both help soothe anxiety and their spicy, earthy scents pair well with bay laurel's herbal aroma; pine and rosemary also help relax tense muscles; ginger offers added circulation support.

What is it?: Bay leaves, from the *Laurus nobilis* tree, are found in kitchens all around the world, and are steam distilled to create bay laurel essential oil.

This slightly sweet herbal oil can treat a range of ailments from dandruff to digestive issues.

Be safe: Do not use bay laurel internally. It may irritate sensitive skin, so do a patch test before using. Do not use bay laurel while pregnant or breastfeeding.

TRY IT OUT:

 Bath: For a bath that supports drainage of the lymph nodes, and also boosts circulation, add 4 drops of bay laurel and 2 drops of ginger to a tablespoon of a carrier oil and add to a warm bath.

 Massage: For an uplifting rub that will ease muscle pain, create a massage oil. Add 12 drops of bay laurel and 6 drops of rosemary to 2 tablespoons (30ml) of a carrier oil (scale up as needed). Blend and massage directly into skin in affected area.

 Hair care: To treat dandruff and stimulate follicles for healthy hair, add 4 drops of bay laurel to a single-use amount of shampoo. Massage it into your scalp and wash as usual.

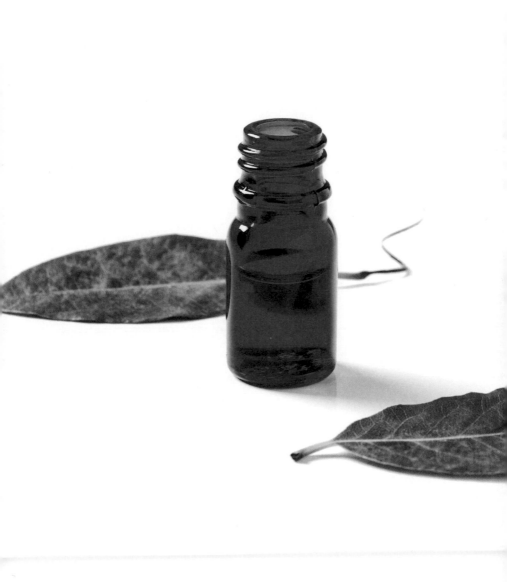

CLARY SAGE

Salvia sclarea

 Use it for: Alleviating anxiety; easing symptoms of PMS or menopause; de-stressing; increasing concentration; boosting libido.

 Blend it with: Geranium and lemongrass enhance clary sage's PMS support; jasmine's floral scent complements its nutty aroma; rose has similar aphrodisiac qualities; tangerine assists with alertness.

What is it?: The leaves and flowering tops of *Salvia sclarea*, a tall biennial herb with blossoms in shades of purple, pink, and white, are distilled to create clary sage essential oil. It has an earthy, herbal scent with calming and anti-inflammatory benefits.

Be safe: Do not use clary sage while pregnant or breastfeeding.

TRY IT OUT:

 Bath: To combat menstrual symptoms from irritability to muscle cramps, add 7 drops of clary sage to a tablespoon of a carrier oil and add to a warm bath.

 Diffusion: Diffuse clary sage in the home to create a calm environment.

 Indirect inhalation: For an on-the-go anxiety aid, create an aromatic spritzer. Add 12 drops of clary sage, 10 drops of sandalwood, and 8 drops of jasmine to ¼ cup (50ml) water in a small, portable amber or dark blue spray bottle. To use, spray in the air and walk through it, inhaling deeply.

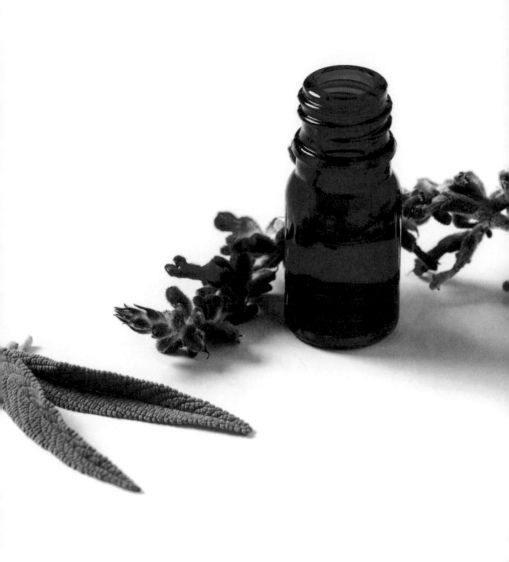

DILL SEED

Anethum graveolens

 Use it for: Supporting digestion, alleviating gas, soothing headaches, easing anxiety, supporting detoxification.

 Blend it with: Nutmeg and spearmint are also great for treating indigestion; lemon complements with immune-boosting properties; elemi also promotes relaxation; fennel has similar detoxification benefits.

What is it?: *Anethum graveolens* is one of the world's most popular culinary herbs, better known as dill. The seeds of this flowering herb, which features thin, delicate leaves, are steam distilled to create dill seed oil. It has a fresh, grass-like scent and is as beneficial in your personal apothecary as it is in your kitchen.

Be safe: Do not use dill seed while pregnant or breastfeeding. Dill seed oil is a photosensitizer; do not use on skin that may be exposed to the sun.

TRY IT OUT:

 Bath: A dill seed oil bath is both relaxing and cleansing. Add 3 drops of dill seed to a tablespoon of a carrier oil and add to a warm bath.

 Diffusion: Create a relaxing, supportive environment by diffusing dill seed. This diffusion can also help with gastrointestinal issues.

 Massage: To target symptoms of indigestion, create a massage oil. Add 10 to 15 drops of dill seed to 2 tablespoons (30ml) of a carrier oil. Blend and massage directly onto your abdomen.

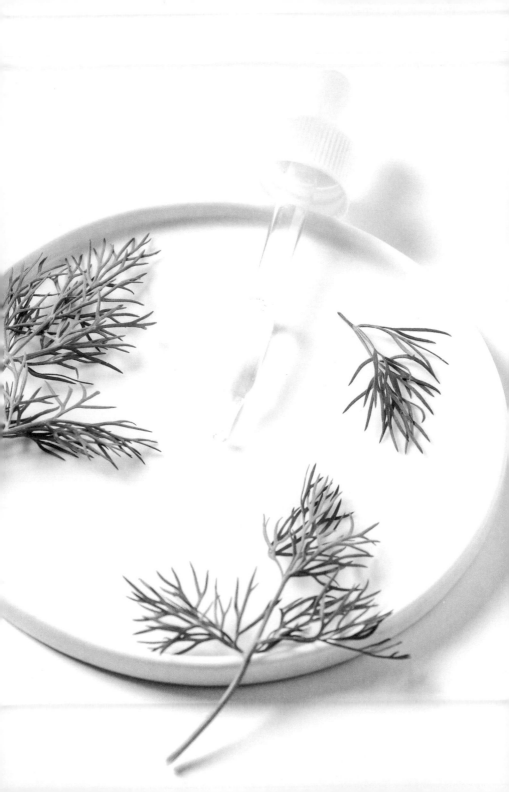

FENNEL

Foeniculum vulgare

 Use it for: Aiding digestion, supporting detoxification, treating problem skin, regulating the menstrual cycle, mitigating symptoms of PMS.

 Blend it with: Cardamom and peppermint also soothe digestive issues; cypress and grapefruit have similar detoxifying properties; the citrus aroma of bergamot pairs well with fennel's sweet herbaceous scent.

What is it?: The seeds of *Foeniculum vulgare*, a flowering herb with delicate leaves, are dried and steam distilled to create fennel essential oil. The warm oil has a sweet, strong licorice scent and is used for treating a range of issues from skin irritations to indigestion.

Be safe: Do not use fennel internally. Do not use fennel while pregnant or breastfeeding. If you have epilepsy or are prone to seizures, refrain from use.

TRY IT OUT:

 Bath: For a detoxifying bath that can also boost self-esteem, add 6 drops of fennel to a tablespoon of a carrier oil and add to a warm bath.

 Skincare: To treat oily skin and blemish flare-ups, add 1 drop of fennel and a couple of drops of witch hazel to a cotton ball and swipe over your face, or the problem areas, after cleansing.

 Direct application: When feeling bloated, gassy, or uneasy in the gut, create a hot compress by mixing 6 drops of fennel and 2 drops of cardamom in a cup of hot water. Take a clean, folded facecloth and place it on top of the water, letting it soak up as much oil and water as possible. Wring out the water and place the compress on your abdomen.

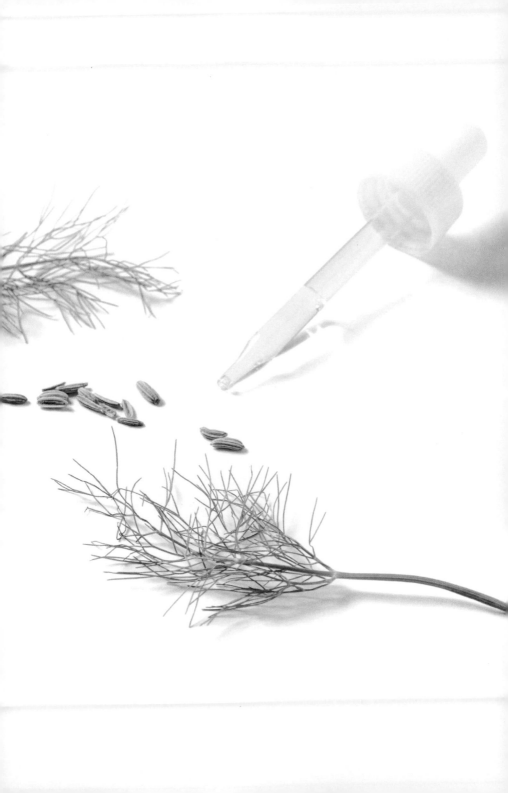

HYSSOP

Hyssopus officinalis

 Use it for: Treating a sore throat, soothing chest congestion, addressing respiratory issues, relieving fatigue, preventing infection.

 Blend it with: Basil also has infection-fighting properties; grapefruit and rosemary can help increase alertness; lemon can also treat a sore throat; lavender adds a nice floral scent to hyssop's herbaceous aroma.

What is it?: *Hyssopus officinalis* is a bushy herb whose leaves and purple flowering tops are steam distilled to create hyssop essential oil. Hyssop was a medicinal mainstay in ancient Greece and was used during biblical times to cleanse temples. Add this oil, which has a subtly sweet, camphoraceous scent, to your own collection for its ability to help you breathe easy, physically and emotionally.

Be safe: Do not use hyssop internally. Do not use hyssop while pregnant or breastfeeding. If you have epilepsy or are prone to seizures, refrain from use.

TRY IT OUT:

 Bath: Tap into hyssop's long history as an oil of purification by adding 3 drops of hyssop and 2 drops of lavender to a tablespoon of a carrier oil and add to a warm bath.

 Steam inhalation: To ease a sore throat and congestion from a cold, add 3 to 5 drops of hyssop to a bowl of hot water. Place a towel over your head, lean over the bowl, and inhale deeply for a minute or two.

 Direct application: Reap hyssop's respiratory benefits along with its aromatherapeutic properties by creating a chest liniment: mix 7 drops of hyssop and 3 drops of rosemary with several drops of a carrier oil. Use your fingers to apply directly to your chest and inhale deeply.

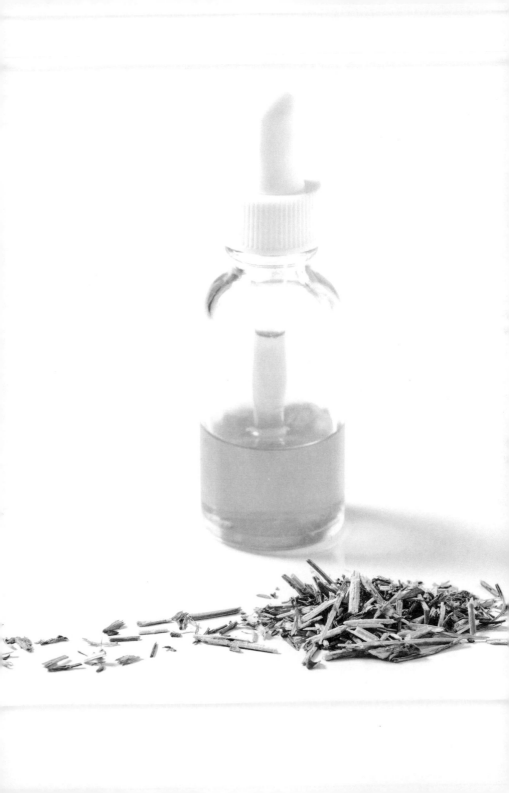

LEMONGRASS

Cymbopogon flexuosus

 Use it for: Fighting infection, repelling insects, supporting detoxification, treating blemishes, boosting skin health, energizing the mind.

 Blend it with: Geranium also supports healthy skin; tea tree boosts its antibacterial properties; citronella and peppermint help repel insects; patchouli enhances its mindfulness effect.

What is it?: The slender leaves of *Cymbopogon flexuosus*, a grass native to Asia, are steam distilled to extract lemongrass essential oil. This essence has a citrus-forward scent with a hint of earthiness. It also has a wide range of benefits, from its antibacterial properties to its analgesic effects.

Be safe: Lemongrass may irritate sensitive skin, so do a patch test before using. Do not use lemongrass while pregnant or breastfeeding.

TRY IT OUT:

 Bath: For a detoxifying bath that can also boost your mental clarity, add 5 to 8 drops of lemongrass to a tablespoon of a carrier oil and add to a warm bath.

 Direct inhalation: For a quick and easy way to break through a mental fog, rub 1 drop of lemongrass between your palms, place hands over your nose, and inhale deeply.

 Skincare: To create a blemish-battling face wash, mix ½ cup (120ml) of an unscented castile soap with 2 tablespoons of jojoba oil and 10 drops of lemongrass. Shake before each use.

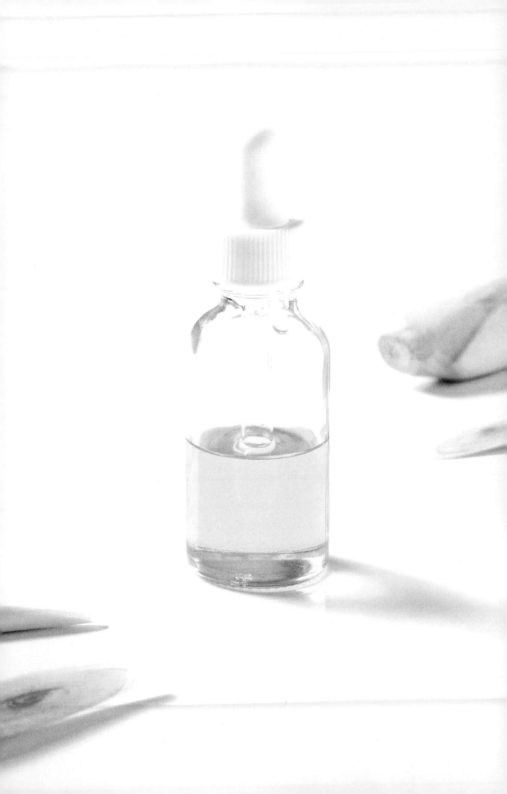

MELISSA

Melissa officinalis

 Use it for: Treating intestinal issues, easing symptoms of PMS, combating viral infections, calming the mind, boosting skin health.

 Blend it with: Lavender enhances its sleep-supporting properties; bergamot and Roman chamomile amp up its soothing effect; sweet orange adds uplift to melissa's stress reduction; geranium rounds out its skin benefits.

What is it?: The leaves and flowers of *Melissa officinalis*, a bushy herb with small white blossoms, are steam distilled to create melissa essential oil, also known as lemon balm. It has a soft citrus, slightly herbaceous scent and is known for its antiviral properties as well as its emotionally calming benefits.

Be safe: Melissa may irritate sensitive skin, so do a patch test before using. Do not use melissa while pregnant or breastfeeding.

TRY IT OUT:

 Bath: For a soothing bath that will prep you for a good night's sleep, add 3 drops of melissa, 2 drops of lavender, and 1 drop of Roman chamomile to a tablespoon of a carrier oil and add to a warm bath.

 Direct application: For those prone to cold sores, melissa can be a powerful healing treatment. Dilute a couple of drops of of melissa with a few drops of water and use a cotton swab to apply directly to the affected area, as soon as you feel the onset of a cold sore. Repeat several times a day.

 Compress: To alleviate the discomfort of menstrual cramps, create a hot compress by mixing 8 drops of melissa in 1 cup (250ml) hot water. Place a clean, folded facecloth on top of the water, letting it soak up as much oil and water as possible. Wring out and place the compress on your abdomen.

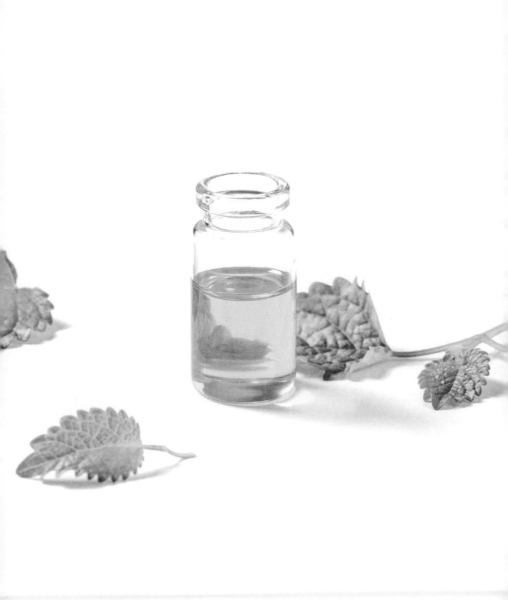

OREGANO

Origanum vulgare

 Use it for: Warding off viruses, alleviating cold and flu symptoms, boosting the immune system, treating infections, cleaning the house.

 Blend it with: Lemon and grapefruit boost its antibacterial qualities; eucalyptus and rosemary also help treat chest congestion; the floral scent of petitgrain softens oregano's herbaceous bite.

What is it?: The leaves of this common household herb, *Origanum vulgare*, are steam distilled to create oregano essential oil. This intensely herbaceous-smelling oil is "hot" and potent, so remember that a little goes a long way toward taking advantage of its antiseptic, antiviral, and pain-soothing qualities. Always dilute this oil with a carrier oil.

Be safe: Oregano may irritate sensitive skin, so do a patch test before using. Do not use oregano while pregnant or breastfeeding.

TRY IT OUT:

 Diffusion: To ward off illness during cold and flu season, or to mitigate symptoms if you're already sick, diffuse a blend of oregano, rosemary, and eucalyptus.

 Home: Oregano's antibacterial qualities make it great for cleaning. To make a spray for kitchen worktops, mix 1 cup (250ml) of vinegar with 5 cups (1250ml) water in a spray bottle. Add 10 drops of oregano, 4 drops of lemon, and 2 drops of grapefruit. Shake to combine.

 Direct application: Take advantage of oregano's antimicrobial properties to treat athlete's foot. Mix 2 to 3 drops of oregano in a tablespoon of a carrier oil and rub on the affected area. Cover with a sock and wash your hands thoroughly.

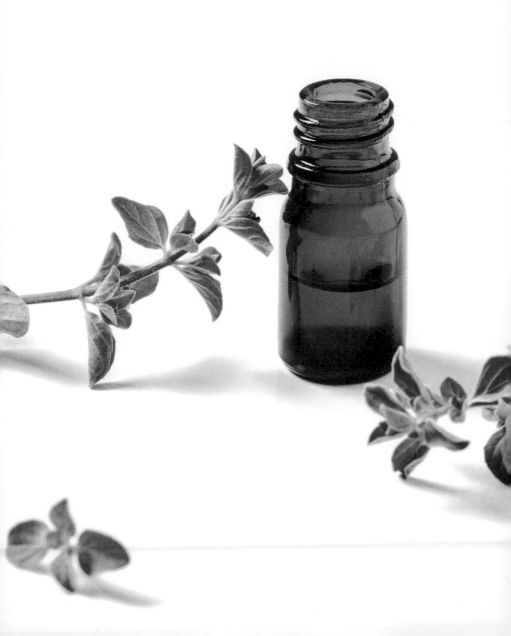

SAGE

Salvia officinalis

 Use it for: Treating stiff muscles, alleviating the symptoms of PMS, repelling insects, soothing dry skin, rejuvenating mentally.

 Blend it with: Rosemary and thyme also ease muscle tension; lavender's scent and soothing qualities complement sage's properties; lemon boosts its antiseptic quality; melissa helps refresh skin.

What is it?: The leaves of *Salvia officinalis*, a shrub-like herb in the mint family, are steam distilled to create sage essential oil. This essence has long been used in apothecaries, and the medicinal and herbaceous oil can be used for a number of healing treatments.

Be safe: Sage may irritate sensitive skin, so do a patch test before using. Do not use sage internally. If you have epilepsy or are prone to seizures, refrain from use. People with high blood pressure should avoid using it. Do not use sage while pregnant or breastfeeding.

TRY IT OUT:

 Direct application: To create an insect repellent, mix 2 tablespoons (30ml) water and 2 tablespoons (30ml) of witch hazel in a small spray bottle. Add 10 drops of sage, 6 drops of lemongrass, and 4 drops of lavender and shake to blend. Spray on your clothes and skin as needed.

 Shower: Use your morning shower to take advantage of sage's stimulating effect. After washing, with the hot water still running, apply 3 drops of sage to a facecloth and rub it over your body, inhaling deeply as you do so.

 Compress: To treat muscle tension, create a hot compress by mixing 8 drops of sage in 1 cup (250ml) hot water. Place a clean, folded facecloth on top of the water, letting it soak up as much oil and water as possible. Wring out the water and place the compress on the affected area.

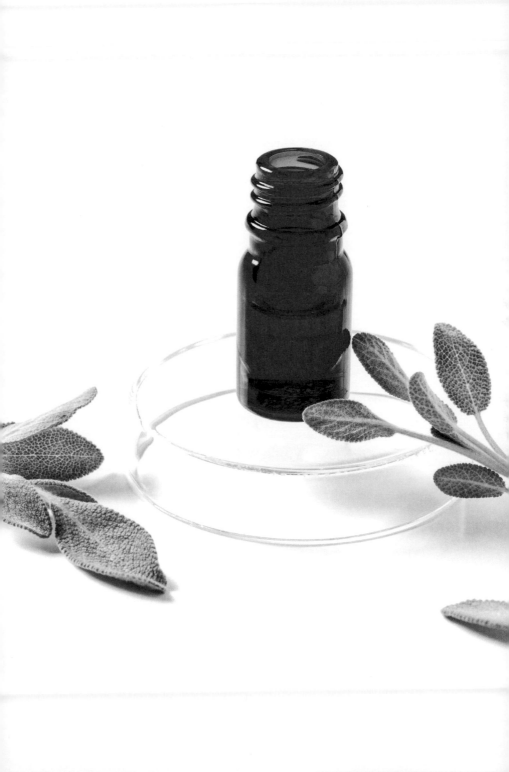

SWEET MARJORAM

Origanum majorana

 Use it for: Enhancing a sense of well-being, treating respiratory issues, soothing inflamed muscles, supporting circulation, alleviating symptoms of PMS and menopause.

 Blend it with: German chamomile boosts its calming effect; eucalyptus and peppermint enhance its respiratory benefits; bergamot and sweet orange add an energizing aroma to marjoram's herbaceous scent.

What is it?: *Origanum majorana* is a fragrant, bushy herb with small green leaves and stems topped with clusters of white or purple flowers. The blooming tops and leaves are steam distilled to create marjoram essential oil, which has a spicy, herbaceous aroma. Marjoram is a culinary staple, but the essential oil has benefits for mood boosting and pain relief, too.

Be safe: Sweet marjoram ay cause drowsiness. Do not use sweet marjoram while pregnant or breastfeeding.

TRY IT OUT:

 Diffusion: Sweet marjoram's ability to promote calm makes it perfect for diffusion—use it at home to put yourself and your guests at ease.

 Steam inhalation: To ease chest congestion caused by a cold or allergies, add 3 to 5 drops of sweet marjoram to a bowl of hot water. Place a towel over your head, lean over the bowl, and inhale deeply for a minute or two.

 Direct application: Take advantage of sweet marjoram's analgesic properties by rubbing it onto sore, stiff muscles. Mix a few drops of sweet marjoram with a few drops of a carrier oil and massage into tender areas.

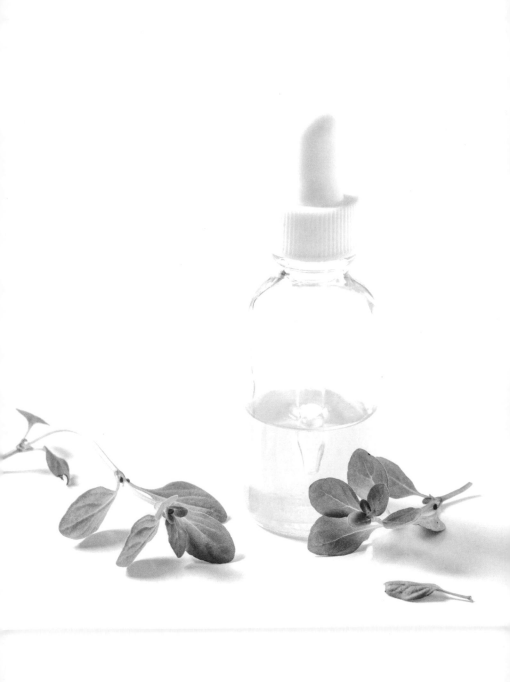

TAGETES

Tagetes minuta

 Use it for: Repelling insects, treating fungal infections, softening corns and calluses, alleviating congestion.

 Blend it with: Citronella and grapefruit are also helpful insect repellents; lemon boosts its antifungal properties; blue chamomile helps soften skin; clary sage gives tagetes's floral scent an earthy grounding.

What is it?: Tagetes essential oil is distilled from the leaves and flowers of *Tagetes minuta*, a tall plant with small yellow-orange blooms native to South America. It is also known as the southern marigold and has a sweet, earthy scent with floral, citrus, and herbaceous notes. It is a very powerful essence, so be sure to dilute it when you are taking advantage of its various benefits, from deterring insects to treating skin issues.

Be safe: Tagetes may irritate sensitive skin, so do a patch test before using. Do not use tagetes while pregnant or breastfeeding. Tagetes is a photosensitizer; do not use on skin that may be exposed to the sun.

TRY IT OUT:

 Diffusion: If you're suffering from a cold or are experiencing chest congestion, diffuse tagetes in the home to help open your lungs.

 Bath: To address foot issues, such as corns and calluses, try this foot bath: add 3 drops of tagetes and 5 drops of blue chamomile to a tablespoon of a carrier oil and mix into a large bowl of warm water. Soak your feet, massaging the oil into the skin with your fingers for 5 to 10 minutes.

 Direct application: To treat athlete's foot, mix 1 drop of tagetes and 2 drops of lemon in a tablespoon of a carrier oil. Blend and apply directly to your affected foot.

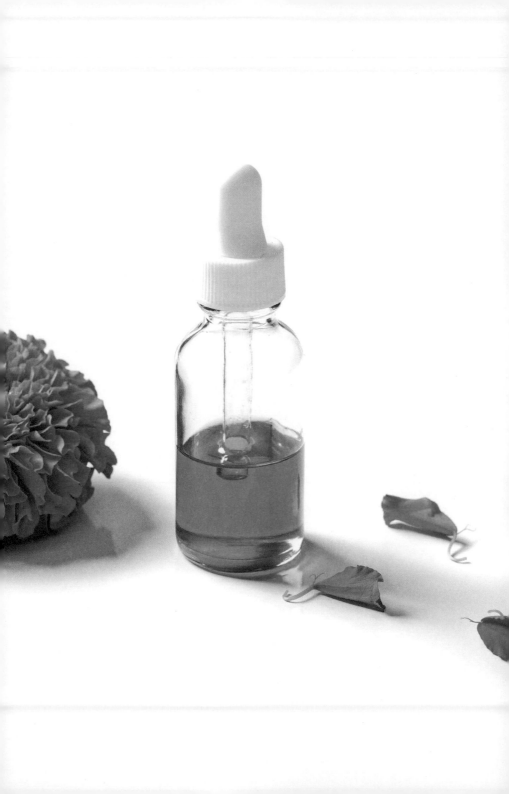

THYME

Thymus vulgaris

 Use it for: Improving concentration, relaxing stiff muscles, supporting the immune system, alleviating cold symptoms, treating blemished skin.

 Blend it with: Lavender boosts thyme's calming nature; ginger also aids in muscle pain relief; tea tree can help ward off sickness; eucalyptus and rosemary ease congestion.

What is it?: The small green leaves and pink, white, or purple flowers of *Thymus vulgaris*, a fragrant, bushy herb, are steam distilled to create thyme essential oil. The herb is a culinary mainstay, but this "hot" herbaceous oil has antiseptic and analgesic qualities as well, and can also be both physically and mentally stimulating.

Be safe: Thyme may irritate sensitive skin, so do a patch test before using. Do not use thyme while pregnant or breastfeeding.

TRY IT OUT:

 Massage: For a warm and soothing back massage, try this blended oil. Add 20 drops of thyme and 10 drops of lavender to ⅓ cup (75ml) of a carrier oil. Blend and massage directly into the back, particularly into any sore areas.

 Steam inhalation: To ease sinus congestion, add 3 drops of thyme and 2 drops of eucalyptus oil to a bowl of hot water. Place a towel over your head, lean over the bowl, and inhale deeply for a minute or two.

 Skincare: Thyme's antibacterial properties make it useful for treating acne-prone skin. Create a toner by adding 6 drops of thyme to 2 tablespoons (30ml) of witch hazel in a small amber or dark blue bottle. To use, shake to blend, dab onto a cotton ball, and wipe over the blemish-prone areas of your face after cleansing.

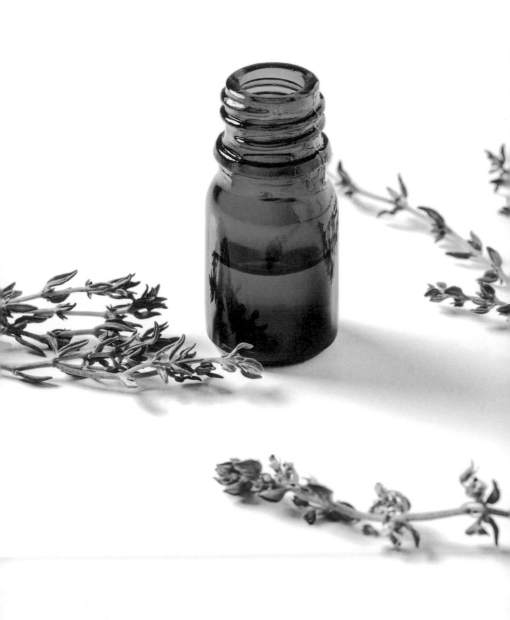

YARROW

Achillea millefolium

 Use it for: Smoothing skin, alleviating congestion, easing menstrual cramps, soothing sore muscles, calming the mind.

 Blend it with: Roman chamomile and blue chamomile enhance its soothing properties; atlas cedarwood can help ground emotions; geranium has similar skin-boosting qualities; rosemary will help ease sore muscles while also stimulating circulation.

What is it?: The small, daisy-like flowers of the herb *Achillea millefolium* are steam distilled to create yarrow essential oil. An anti-inflammatory for the body and a de-stressor for the mind, this calming oil has a subtle earthy, herbaceous scent with a hint of fruitiness.

Be safe: Yarrow may irritate sensitive skin, so do a patch test before using. Do not use yarrow while pregnant or breastfeeding.

TRY IT OUT:

 Compress: To alleviate the discomfort of menstrual cramps, create a hot compress by mixing 10 drops of yarrow in 1 cup (250ml) hot water. Take a clean, folded facecloth and place it on top of the water, letting it soak up as much oil and water as possible. Wring out the water and place the compress on your abdomen.

 Massage: For sore muscle relief, create a massage oil. Add 10 to 15 drops of yarrow to 2 tablespoons (30ml) of a carrier oil (scale up as needed). Blend and massage directly into the skin.

 Steam inhalation: To ease congestion, add 3 to 5 drops of yarrow to a bowl of hot water. Place a towel over your head, lean over the bowl, and inhale deeply for a minute or two.

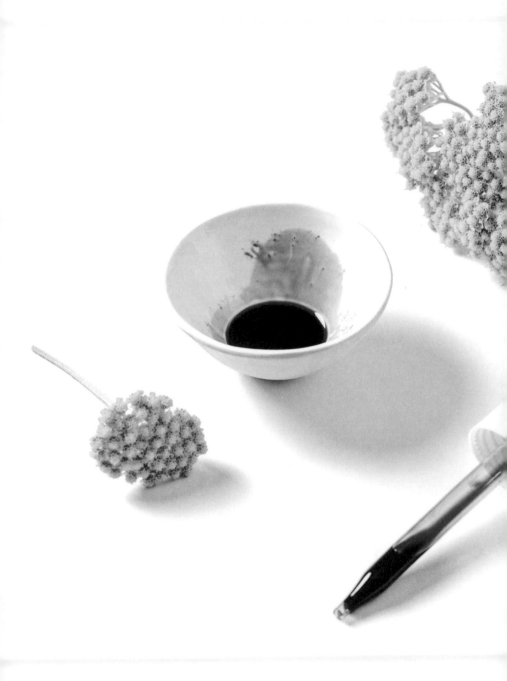

CAJEPUT

Melaleuca leucadendra

 Use it for: Repelling insects, soothing a sore throat, clearing sinuses, treating problem skin, reenergizing.

 Blend it with: Pine or peppermint boosts its decongesting properties; clove is also an insect repellent; lemon increases its antiseptic benefits; sandalwood can help soothe a sore throat.

What is it?: Leaves and twigs of the *Melaleuca leucadendra*, a tall tree with a flaky white bark, are steam distilled to create cajeput essential oil, which has a medicinal smell reminiscent of eucalyptus, with a subtle hint of fruitiness. It's lesser known than its camphoraceous counterparts but has many of the same benefits, from treating cold symptoms to offering a mental pick-me-up.

Be safe: Cajeput may irritate sensitive skin, so do a patch test before using.

TRY IT OUT:

 Mouth care: To ease the pain of a sore throat and aid in recovery, try gargling with cajeput. Mix 1 drop of cajeput and 1 drop of sandalwood in 2 tablespoons (30ml) water. Gargle, then spit it out.

 Shower: To combat the congestion and exhaustion of a cold, try showering with cajeput to help clear your mind and your chest. After washing, with the hot water still running, apply 3 drops of cajeput to a facecloth and rub it over your body, inhaling deeply as you do so.

 Skincare: To treat blemishes and prevent breakouts, add 1 drop of cajeput to a single-use amount of your daily facial cleanser before applying. Wash and rinse as usual.

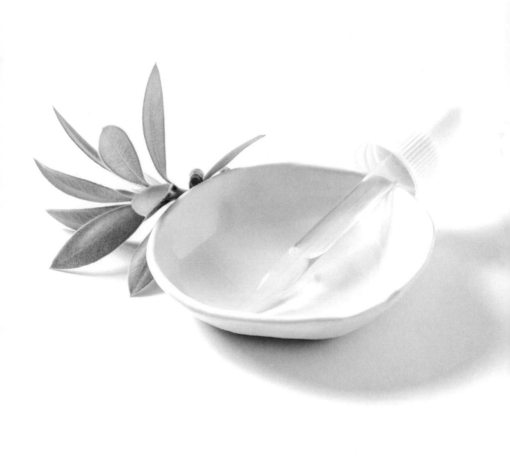

EUCALYPTUS

Eucalyptus globulus

 Use it for: Alleviating respiratory issues, easing sore muscles, aiding mental clarity, increasing relaxation, cleaning the home.

 Blend it with: Lavender boosts its relaxing effects; lemon and tea tree enhance its antibacterial properties; peppermint helps clear chest congestion; rosemary complements the soothing of muscles.

What is it?: It's the long, thin leaves and twigs of the blue gum, or *Eucalyptus globulus*, a tall tree native to Australia, that are steam distilled to create eucalyptus essential oil.

The clean, camphoraceous scent is centering, and eucalyptus oil has a number of benefits for easing cold and flu symptoms.

Be safe: Do not use eucalyptus internally. Do not use eucalyptus while pregnant or breastfeeding.

TRY IT OUT:

 Home: Reap the antibacterial and antiseptic benefits of eucalyptus with this floor cleaner: mix 1 cup (250ml) of white vinegar into 1 gallon (4 liters) hot water and add 20 drops of eucalyptus. Use the mixture to mop.

 Massage: For a massage that will target sore muscles and leave you feeling relaxed but alert, create a massage oil. Add 10 drops of eucalyptus, 8 drops of rosemary, and 6 drops of lavender to ¼ cup (50ml) of a carrier oil. Blend and massage directly into skin.

 Steam inhalation: To ease chest and/or sinus congestion, add 3 to 5 drops of eucalyptus to a bowl of hot water. Place a towel over your head, lean over the bowl, and inhale deeply for a minute or two.

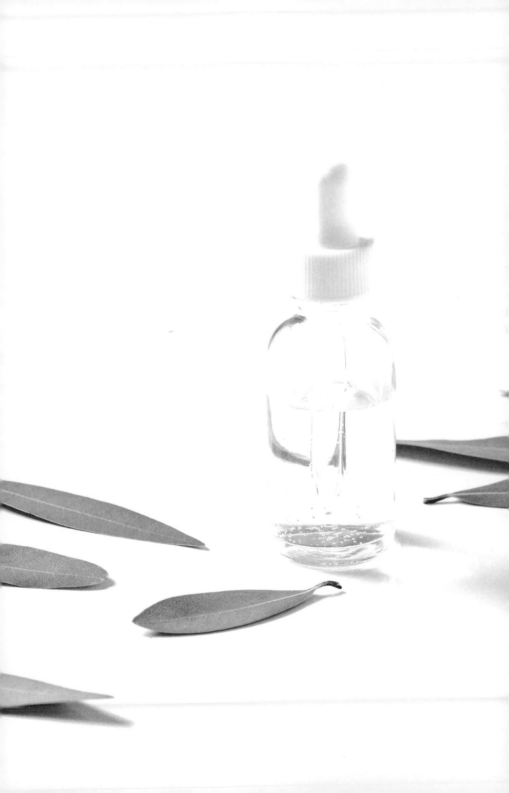

NIAOULI

Melaleuca viridiflora

 Use it for: Healing cuts and scrapes, fighting infection, supporting the immune system, easing congestion, treating blemishes.

 Blend it with: Eucalyptus and tea tree are also strong decongestants; lemon can help boost immunity; rosemary increases its antibacterial qualities; sweet orange adds an uplifting citrus zing to niaouli's fatigue-fighting camphoraceous scent.

What is it?: *Melaleuca viridiflora* is a tree with peeling bark and white bottlebrush flowers. Its leaves and twigs are steam distilled to create the antiseptic, antibacterial niaouli oil, which has a strong medicinal scent with a touch of sweetness.

Be safe: There are no known precautions associated with niaouli oil.

TRY IT OUT:

 Diffusion: Support your health during cold and flu season by diffusing niaouli in the home.

 Skincare: Niaouli has similar bacteria-fighting properties to tea tree oil but is less potent and more suitable for those with sensitive skin. Try it in a clarifying toner: in a small amber or dark blue bottle, mix ¼ cup (50ml) of water with 1 tablespoons (15ml) of apple cider vinegar and 6 drops of niaouli. Using a cotton pad, swipe the mixture over your cleansed face.

 Steam inhalation: To help lessen the severity of a cold or the flu, add 3 to 5 drops of niaouli to a bowl of hot water. Place a towel over your head, lean over the bowl, and inhale deeply for a minute or two.

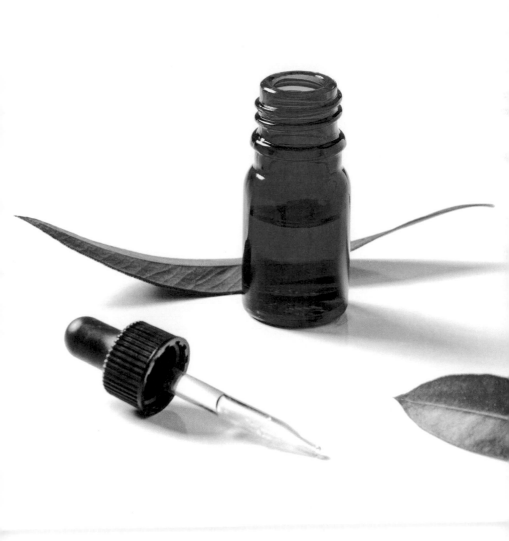

PEPPERMINT

Mentha x piperita

 Use it for: Alleviating foot odor, quelling the pain and itchiness of insect bites, rejuvenating mentally, boosting energy, cooling a fever.

 Blend it with: Eucalyptus boosts its analgesic qualities; frankincense is also anti-itch; lavender's soothing properties complement peppermint's cooling attributes; sweet orange and rosemary complement its scent and ability to reinvigorate.

What is it?: Peppermint essential oil is steam distilled from *Mentha* x *piperita*, an aromatic plant with small, dark green leaves and tiny pink or purple flower blossoms. This fresh, minty oil is both analgesic and antimicrobial, and has energizing qualities, making it a go-to for novice and experienced oil users alike.

Be safe: Peppermint may irritate sensitive skin, so do a patch test before using. Do not use peppermint while pregnant or breastfeeding.

TRY IT OUT:

 Direct inhalation: For a quick pick-me-up, rub 1 drop of peppermint between your palms, place hands over your nose, and inhale deeply.

 Direct application: To help treat foot odor, create a foot/shoe spray. In a small amber or dark blue spray bottle, add 10 drops of peppermint to ¼ cup (50ml) of rubbing alcohol. Shake well and spray in shoes daily, and on feet after showering.

 Direct application: To alleviate the itch of insect bites, dilute 1 drop of peppermint and 1 drop of lavender with a couple of drops of a carrier oil. Use your finger to dab it directly on a bite.

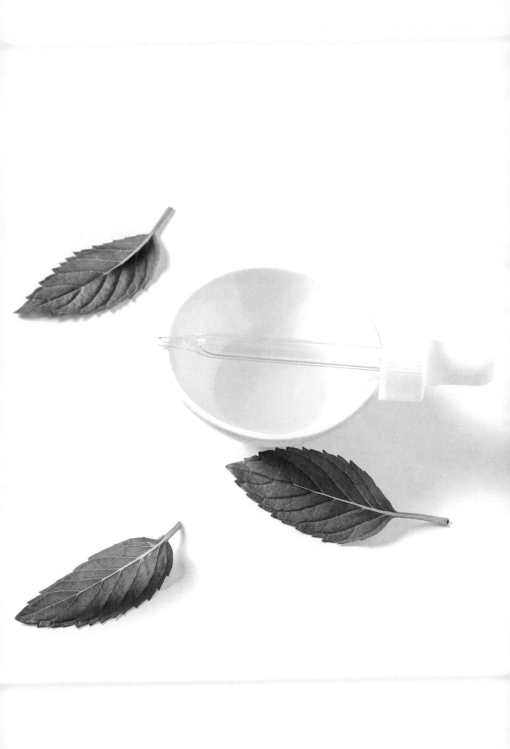

ROSEMARY

Rosmarinus officinalis

 Use it for: Improving circulation, boosting alertness, soothing tense muscles, alleviating headaches, cleaning the house.

 Blend it with: Peppermint boosts rosemary's energizing properties; lavender and sage help promote muscle relaxation; lemon and grapefruit are also great for house cleaning.

What is it?: The flowering tops of *Rosmarinus officinalis*, a spiky, bushy herb widely used in kitchens around the world, are steam distilled to create rosemary essential oil. This slightly sweet- and medicinal-smelling oil is incredibly versatile, with energy- and mood-boosting benefits, analgesic qualities, and antibacterial properties that make it an effective element in household cleaning products.

Be safe: Do not use rosemary while pregnant or breastfeeding. If you have epilepsy or are prone to seizures, refrain from use.

TRY IT OUT:

 Home: For extra antibacterial and antiseptic qualities, add rosemary to unscented liquid hand soap, about 1 to 2 drops per ¼ to ⅓ cup (50–75ml).

 Massage: To soothe muscle pain or mitigate muscle spasms, create a massage oil. Add 7 drops of rosemary and 5 drops of lavender to 2 tablespoons (30ml) of a carrier oil (scale up as needed). Blend and massage directly into the skin.

 Hair care: In addition to improving circulation, rosemary oil stimulates hair follicles. To boost growth or treat dry, unhealthy hair, add 1 to 2 drops of rosemary to a single-use amount of shampoo before applying it to hair and washing as usual.

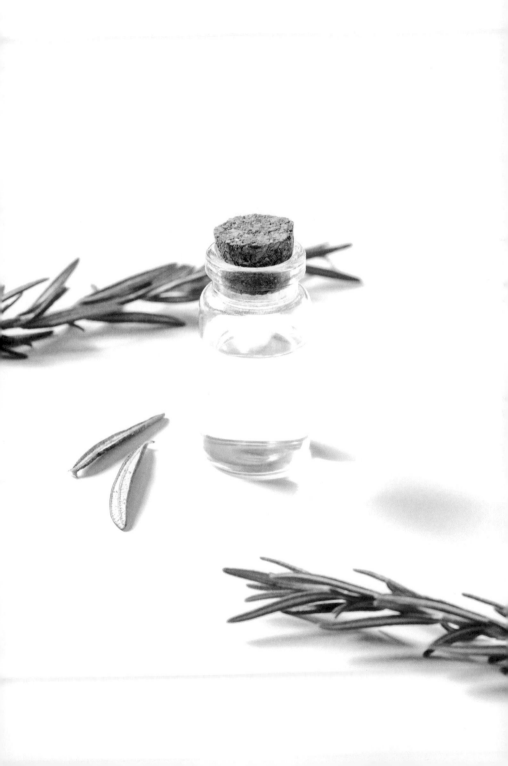

SPEARMINT

Mentha spicata

 Use it for: Freshening breath, easing nausea, soothing indigestion, treating congestion, cleaning the home.

 Blend it with: Lemon and rosemary increase its antiseptic and antibacterial properties; eucalyptus increases spearmint's effectiveness as a decongestant; sweet orange adds a lovely citrus scent to spearmint's refreshing freshness.

What is it?: The aromatic leaves of the flowering herb *Mentha spicata* are steam distilled to create spearmint essential oil. This sweet, minty oil has many of the same properties as peppermint but with less menthol in its makeup, creating a less abrasive effect. It has many benefits from freshening the breath to refreshing the mind.

Be safe: There are no known precautions associated with spearmint oil.

TRY IT OUT:

 Direct inhalation: To help ease nausea and ground yourself during motion sickness, rub 1 drop of spearmint between your palms, place hands over your nose, and inhale deeply.

 Home: For an antibacterial all-purpose cleaning spray that will also freshen up a room, mix 1 cup (250ml) of vinegar with 1 cup (250ml) water in a spray bottle. Add 15 drops of spearmint and shake to combine.

 Mouth care: For a refreshing natural mouthwash, mix 1 to 2 drops of spearmint into 2 tablespoons (30ml) water and swish it around in your mouth for 30 seconds after brushing your teeth.

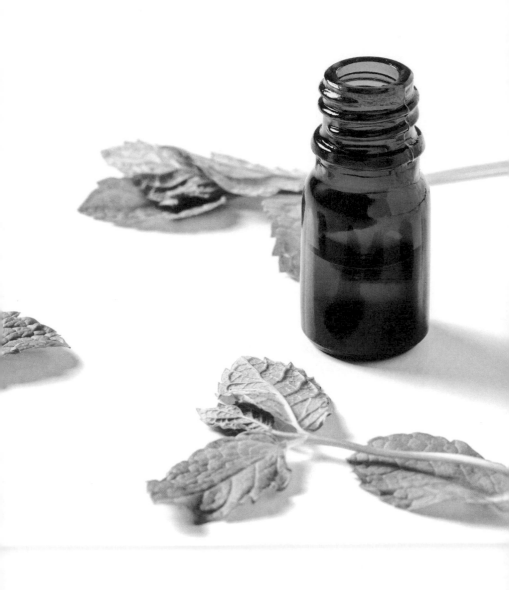

TEA TREE

Melaleuca alternifolia

 Use it for: Treating acne, soothing skin conditions, alleviating dandruff/ itchy scalp, clearing sinuses, cleaning the house.

 Blend it with: The earthy scent of clary sage pairs well with tea tree; eucalyptus has complementary congestion-clearing benefits; the floral scent of lavender softens tea tree's medicinal scent; lemon and ylang-ylang boost its antibacterial properties.

What is it?: Tea tree essential oil is steam distilled from the leaves and twigs of the *Melaleuca alternifolia*, a bushy tree or shrub native to Australia. Because of its antiseptic, antifungal, and anti-inflammatory properties, camphoraceous-scented tea tree oil has a wide range of benefits and uses, from skincare to home cleaning solutions.

Be safe: Do not use tea tree internally. Tea tree may irritate sensitive skin, so do a patch test before using.

TRY IT OUT:

 Home: For an all-purpose kitchen cleaner, mix 1 cup (250ml) of vinegar with 1 cup (250ml) water in a spray bottle. Add 10 drops of tea tree and shake to combine. (Refrain from using on granite or marble.)

 Skincare: To spot-treat breakouts, put 1 drop of tea tree in the palm of your hand. Use your ring finger to dab directly on the pimple. Apply at night before going to bed.

 Steam inhalation: To ease sinus congestion, add 3 to 5 drops of tea tree to a bowl of hot water. Place a towel over your head, lean over the bowl, and inhale deeply for a minute or two.

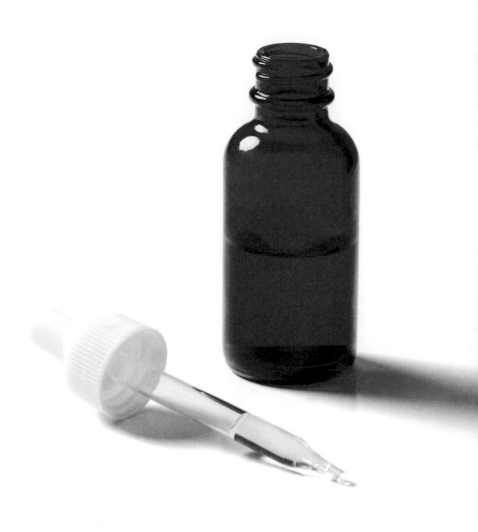

ALLSPICE

Pimenta dioica

Use it for: Easing anxiety, boosting libido, soothing muscle and joint pain, increasing circulation, supporting the digestive system.

Blend it with: Ginger enhances allspice's ability to ease nausea; coriander boosts its benefits to the digestive system; lavender and ylang-ylang add calm and well-being to its grounding effect; sweet orange's bright citrus scent pairs well with allspice's warmth.

What is it?: The small berries of the *Pimenta dioica* tree are steam distilled to create the potent allspice essential oil. The spicy scent—with hints of cinnamon, clove, nutmeg, and pepper—is grounding and calming, and the oil is beneficial for digestive issues and pain as well.

Be safe: Do not use allspice internally. Allspice may irritate sensitive skin, so do a patch test before using.

TRY IT OUT:

Diffusion: Diffuse allspice in the bedroom, especially during the winter months, for a warm, comforting scent that acts as an aphrodisiac.

Massage: Take advantage of allspice's anesthetic and analgesic properties by targeting sore muscles or joints with this massage oil: add 10 drops of allspice to 2 tablespoons (30ml) of a carrier oil and apply directly to skin.

Shower: To wash the stress of the day away and prepare yourself for a good night's sleep, try allspice in your evening shower. After washing, with the hot water still running, apply 3 drops of allspice to a facecloth and rub it over your body, inhaling deeply as you do so.

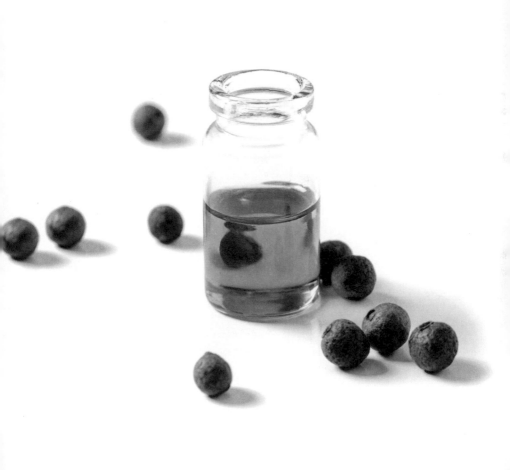

ANISE SEED

Pimpinella anisum

 Use it for: Quelling nausea, easing vertigo, treating indigestion, mitigating bad breath, alleviating respiratory issues.

 Blend it with: Cardamom boosts anise seed's mouth health benefits; coriander has similar nausea-quelling properties; dill seed and fennel are also great for treating indigestion.

What is it?: *Pimpinella anisum* is a tall herb and the seeds of its small white flowers are steam distilled to created anise seed oil. Its spicy, earthy aroma has a note of licorice, and the essence has long been used to treat the symptoms of indigestion.

Be safe: Do not use anise seed internally. Anise seed may irritate sensitive skin, so do a patch test before using. Do not use anise seed while pregnant. Anise seed oil is a photosensitizer; do not use on skin that may be exposed to the sun.

TRY IT OUT:

 Diffusion: When experiencing chest congestion, diffuse anise seed in the home to help open up your airways.

 Direct inhalation: To help combat feelings of nausea, rub 1 drop of anise seed between your palms, place hands over your nose, and inhale deeply.

 Steam inhalation: For relief with bronchitis, add 3 to 5 drops of anise seed to a bowl of hot water. Place a towel over your head, lean over the bowl, and inhale deeply for a minute or two.

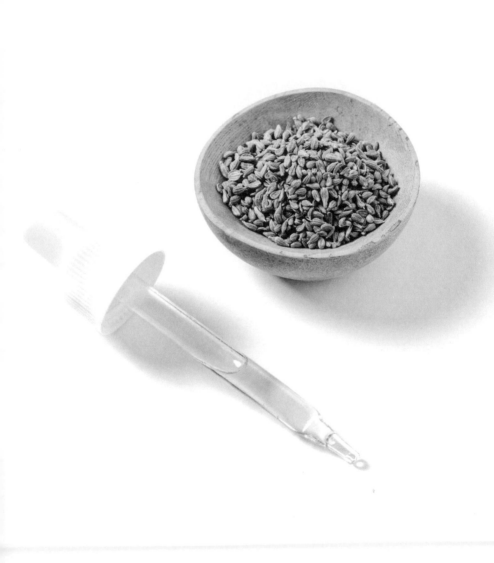

BLACK PEPPER

Piper nigrum

 Use it for: Increasing mental alertness, boosting circulation, enhancing libido, mitigating anxiety, treating indigestion.

 Blend it with: Bergamot and sweet orange add emotional uplift to black pepper's mental stimulation; sandalwood enhances its aphrodisiac effect; ginger helps ease exhaustion and boost circulation.

What is it?: The small fruits of *Piper nigrum*, a flowering vine, are dried and distilled to create black pepper essential oil. Black pepper is one of the most common culinary spices, but its effects as an essential oil are quite different. Though it has a warm, peppery scent, inhaling or diffusing it will not cause sneezing or coughing; instead it offers increased mental acuity as well as a range of physiological benefits.

Be safe: Black pepper may irritate sensitive skin, so do a patch test before using. Do not use black pepper while pregnant or breastfeeding.

TRY IT OUT:

 Diffusion: To ease anxiety while mitigating fatigue, diffuse black pepper in the home. Add sandalwood to increase its aphrodisiac properties or bergamot for a supportive, uplifting environment.

 Direct inhalation: For a quick and easy way to clear your mind, rub 1 drop of black pepper between your palms, place hands over your nose, and inhale deeply.

 Massage: For a warming massage during the colder months, add 10 drops of black pepper to 2 tablespoons (30ml) of a carrier oil (scale up as needed). Blend and rub directly into skin for a massage that will boost circulation and ease anxiety.

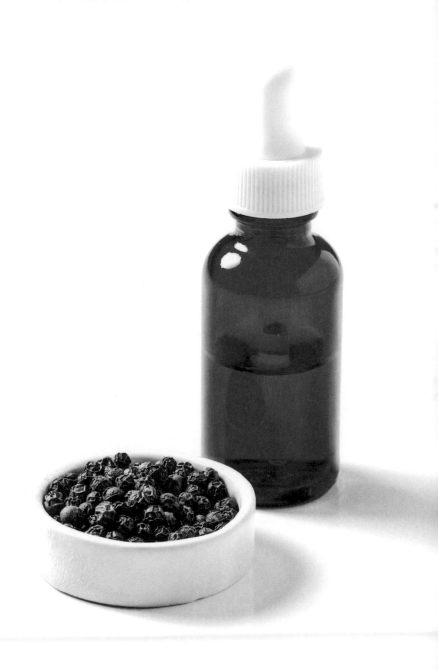

CARAWAY

Carum carvi

Use it for: Supporting digestion, balancing skin, treating an oily scalp, easing nerves, soothing a cough.

Blend it with: Basil can also help balance an oily scalp; blue chamomile and Roman chamomile boost caraway's calming properties; coriander and ginger are also great for treating gastrointestinal issues.

What is it?: The small striped seeds of *Carum carvi*, a plant topped with small white flowers, are distilled to create caraway essential oil. Culinarily used in many cultures, caraway seeds impart the essential oil with a spicy, slightly fruity scent that has a subtle hint of licorice. Caraway oil is particularly helpful in aiding digestion but offers skin and hair benefits as well.

Be safe: Caraway may irritate sensitive skin, so do a patch test before using. Do not use caraway while pregnant or breastfeeding.

TRY IT OUT:

Massage: To soothe an upset stomach, add 5 drops of caraway and 2 drops of coriander to a tablespoon of a carrier oil. Using your fingers, rub the blend on your stomach in a clockwise direction, starting on your right side.

Hair care: To help balance a sebaceous scalp, add 2 drops of caraway and 1 drop of basil to a single-use amount of shampoo; use it to wash and rinse as usual.

Compress: For cramps related to indigestion, create a hot compress by mixing 12 drops of caraway in 1 cup (250ml) hot water. Place a clean, folded facecloth on top of the water, letting it soak up as much oil and water as possible. Wring out and place the compress on your lower abdomen.

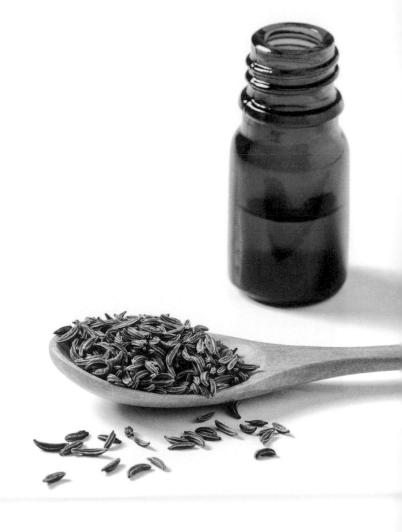

CARDAMOM

Elettaria cardamomum

 Use it for: Boosting mouth health, treating symptoms of indigestion, mitigating nausea, calming skin issues, soothing anxiety.

 Blend it with: Clove helps bust bad breath; cinnamon and nutmeg enhance cardamom's warm, spicy scent; ginger helps quell nausea; petitgrain complements cardamom's soothing effects.

What is it?: Dried fruit or seeds from *Elettaria cardamomum*, an herb native to India, are steam distilled to create cardamom essential oil. This warm, subtle, spicy oil has soothing properties for the mind and the body.

Be safe: There are no known precautions associated with cardamom oil.

TRY IT OUT:

 Mouth care: Add 1 to 2 drops of cardamom to 2 tablespoons (30ml) water. inse with a mouthful whenever you want to freshen your breath.

 Skincare: The scent of cardamom pairs great with coffee. Create a body scrub using ground beans to get the skin-soothing and aromatic benefits, plus a little energy boost. Mix 1 ounce (20g) of ground coffee with 4 ounces (100g) of sugar. Blend 5 to 10 drops of cardamom with 2 tablespoons of carrier oil, then add to the coffee mix and stir. Apply the scrub directly to skin in the shower.

 Direct application: To easily treat or prevent nausea, especially if caused by motion sickness, create this blend to carry with you while traveling. Mix 10 drops of cardamom, 6 drops of ginger, and 4 drops of coriander with 1 tablespoon (15ml) of a carrier oil. Store in an amber or dark blue roller bottle and apply to the inside of your wrists and the back of your neck as needed, inhaling deeply.

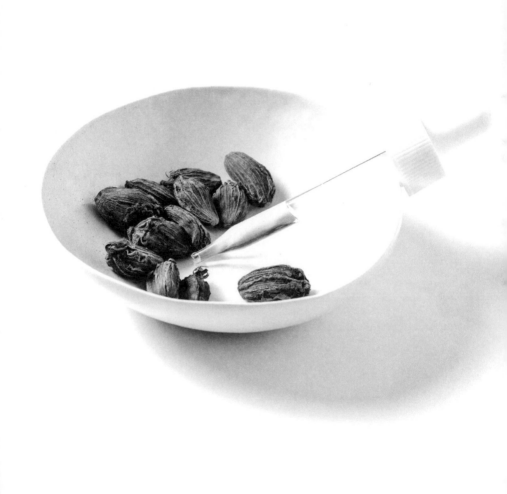

CINNAMON LEAF

Cinnamomum zeylanicum

 Use it for: Curbing sugar cravings, repelling insects, cleaning the home, alleviating exhaustion, relieving pain.

 Blend it with: Ginger can help curb cravings; clove and peppermint boost cinnamon's insect-repelling properties; sweet orange and tangerine add a bright citrus scent and an increased invigoration.

What is it?: The leaves and twigs of *Cinnamomum zeylanicum*, an evergreen tree or shrub, are distilled to create cinnamon leaf essential oil—a gentler essence than cinnamon bark, better suited for the home essential oil user. It has a sweet and spicy scent and offers a number of benefits for the home and for the mind.

Be safe: Cinnamon leaf may irritate sensitive skin, so do a patch test before using. Do not use cinnamon leaf while pregnant or breastfeeding.

TRY IT OUT:

 Direct inhalation: If you're trying to curb a sugar addiction, cinnamon leaf can help. Because cinnamon leaf can be a "hot" oil, rather than rubbing 1 drop between your palms, simply open the bottle, place it under your nose, and inhale deeply.

 Home: Take advantage of cinnamon's antibacterial properties with this bathroom cleaning spray. Mix 1 cup (50ml) water with 1 cup (250ml) of white vinegar and 15 drops of cinnamon leaf. Shake to blend before each use.

 Massage: The spicy-sweet scent of cinnamon leaf oil, combined with its warming properties, makes it perfect for a cold weather massage. Add 8 drops of cinnamon leaf to 2 tablespoons (30ml) of a carrier oil (scale up as needed). Blend and massage directly into skin.

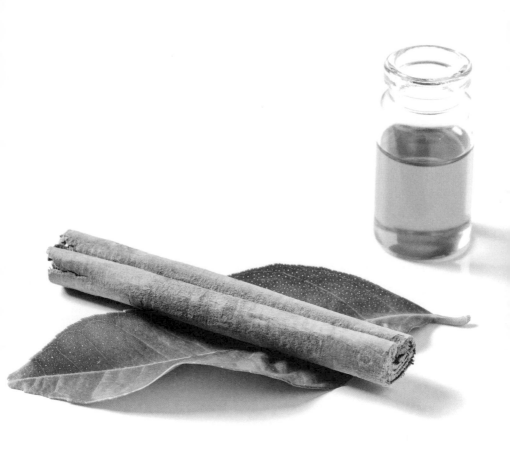

CLOVE

Syzgium aromaticum

 Use it for: Boosting dental health, treating bad breath, alleviating pain, repelling insects, preventing infection.

 Blend it with: Frankincense enhances clove's antiseptic properties; cinnamon and nutmeg complement its warm aroma; benzoin's anti-inflammatory properties pair well with clove's analgesic effect; geranium calms clove's heat.

What is it?: The dried, unopened buds of *Syzygium aromaticum*, a fragrant, leafy tree, have been medicinally used for centuries and are steam distilled to create sweet and spicy clove oil. In addition to its warm, inviting aroma, it has analgesic and anti-inflammatory properties.

Be safe: Don't use clove internally. Don't use it for long periods. Clove may irritate sensitive skin; do a patch test before using. Don't use clove while pregnant or breastfeeding.

TRY IT OUT:

 Mouth care: To treat bad breath and boost overall mouth health, create a rinse by adding 1 drop of clove and 1 drop of tea tree to 2 tablespoons (30ml) water. Swish around in your mouth for 30 seconds after brushing your teeth. Do not swallow.

 Massage: Clove is also known for increasing circulation. Create this foot massage oil to reap its benefits: add 10 drops of geranium and 5 drops of clove to 2 tablespoons (30ml) of a carrier oil (scale up as needed). Blend and massage into feet and lower legs.

 Compress: To alleviate muscle stiffness, create a hot compress by mixing 6 drops of clove in 1 cup (250ml) hot water. Place a clean, folded facecloth on top of the water, letting it soak up as much oil and water as possible. Wring out the water and place the compress on the affected area.

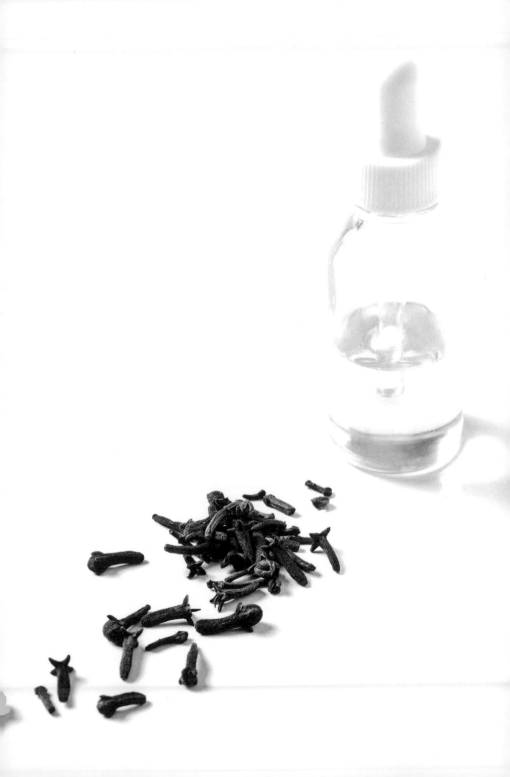

CORIANDER SEED

Coriandrum sativum

 Use it for: Aiding digestion, quelling nausea, soothing stiff muscles, uplifting emotions, balancing oily skin.

 Blend it with: Cardamom and peppermint can help appease symptoms of indigestion; nutmeg also assuages nausea; sweet orange's energizing aroma complements coriander seed's uplift; ylang-ylang's floral scent pairs well with coriander seed's herbaceousness.

What is it?: Seeds from *Coriandrum sativum*, an herb more commonly known as coriander and used in kitchens around the world, are crushed and steam distilled to create coriander seed essential oil. The spicy, herbaceous scent of this oil is also slightly sweet, and its benefits run the gamut from rejuvenating the spirit to relaxing the muscles.

Be safe: Coriander seed may irritate sensitive skin, so do a patch test before using.

TRY IT OUT:

 Massage: After a stressful day, use this massage oil on your neck and shoulders to reenergize. Mix 4 drops of coriander seed, 2 drops of lavender, and 2 drops of sweet orange in 1 tablespoon (15ml) of a carrier oil. Apply to skin.

 Skincare: To treat oily, combination, or acne-prone skin, place a single-use amount of your nightly moisturizer in your palm and add 1 drop of coriander seed before applying to your face.

 Direct application: To treat bloating, gas, and general indigestion, create a rub by mixing 6 drops of coriander seed, 2 drops of peppermint and 2 drops of cardamom into 1 tablespoon (15ml) of a carrier oil. Rub in a clockwise motion on your abdomen.

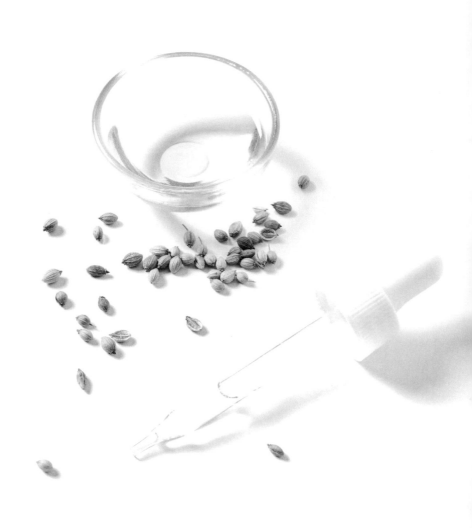

GINGER

Zingiber officinale

 Use it for: Easing motion sickness, treating digestive issues, reducing fever, increasing libido, boosting circulation.

 Blend it with: Allspice enhances its aphrodisiac qualities; cardamom and coriander ease gastrointestinal issues; grapefruit helps quell motion sickness; lime's citrus scent adds a brightness to ginger's warmth.

What is it?: Ginger has been used in kitchens and natural medicine cabinets for centuries, and it is the dried ginger root of *Zingiber officinale*, an herb native to China, that is steam distilled to make this essential oil. Its warm, earthy, spicy scent has a number of benefits, and the oil is used to treat everything from gastrointestinal unease to flu symptoms.

Be safe: Ginger may irritate sensitive skin, so do a patch test before using. Do not use ginger while pregnant or breastfeeding. Ginger oil is a photosensitizer; do not use on skin that may be exposed to the sun.

TRY IT OUT:

 Bath: To ease gastrointestinal ailments, such as bloating, cramps, or gas, take a warm bath with ginger by mixing 3 drops of ginger, 2 drops of cardamom, and 1 drop of cypress into a tablespoon of a carrier oil and add to the bath.

 Diffusion: For a spicy scent that may stoke desire, diffuse ginger along with allspice in the bedroom to create a warm, titillating environment.

 Massage: For a circulation-boosting massage, add 5 drops of ginger, 3 drops of sweet marjoram, and 2 drops of lavender to 2 tablespoons (30ml) of a carrier oil (scale up as needed). Blend and massage directly into skin.

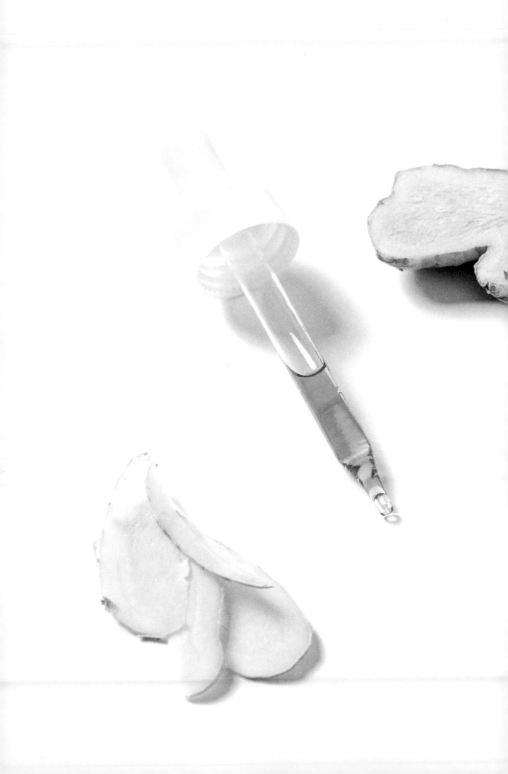

NUTMEG

Myristica fragrans

 Use it for: Quelling nausea and indigestion, alleviating stiff muscles, supporting circulation, mitigating symptoms of PMS.

 Blend it with: The citrus scent of mandarin and sweet orange complement nutmeg's warmth and add an energizing element to its calm; carrot seed and rosemary are similarly soothing.

What is it?: *Myristica fragrans* is an evergreen tree native to Indonesia that produces small flowers and round fruits. The seed of each fruit is dried and steam distilled to create nutmeg essential oil. The warm, slightly sweet and spicy oil is calming and especially helpful for gastrointestinal issues.

Be safe: Do not use nutmeg internally. Do not use nutmeg while pregnant or breastfeeding.

TRY IT OUT:

 Direct inhalation: For a quick remedy to help ease nausea or motion sickness, rub 1 drop of nutmeg between your palms, place hands over your nose, and inhale deeply.

 Diffusion: To enhance an uplifting mood during the winter months, diffuse nutmeg with sweet orange or mandarin for a comforting aroma.

 Direct application: To help relieve bloating, cramps, or other gastrointestinal issues, create a massage oil by adding 10 drops of nutmeg to 2 tablespoons (30 ml) of a carrier oil. Blend and apply directly to your abdomen, rubbing in a gentle clockwise motion.

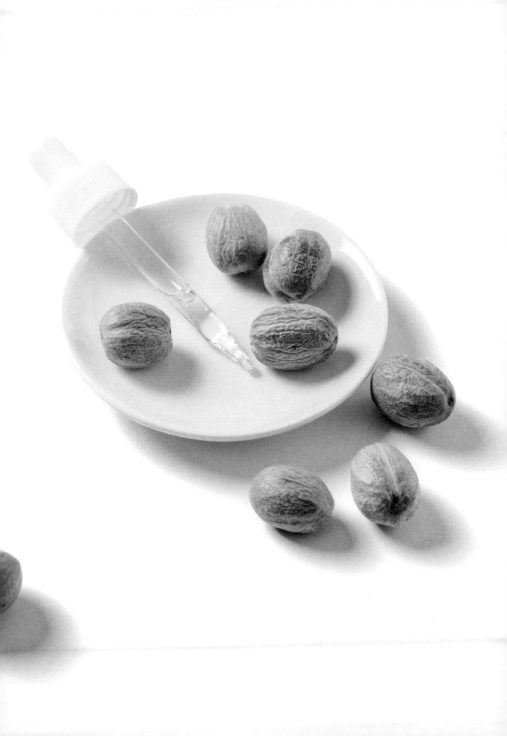

BENZOIN

Styrax tonkinesis

 Use it for: Alleviating insomnia, easing anxiety, relieving cold or flu symptoms, addressing dry skin, treating cuts and scrapes.

 Blend it with: Blue chamomile and sandalwood enhance benzoin's moisturizing properties; the floral scents of jasmine and rose complement benzoin's vanilla notes and emotional effects; ylang-ylang boosts its sleep support.

What is it?: The resin of *Styrax tonkinesis*, a tall, leafy tree with white blossoms, is processed by solvent extraction to produce the thick benzoin essential oil. Its sweet, warm, vanilla-like scent makes benzoin a mainstay in the world of incense and perfume, but its comforting aroma has mental and emotional benefits as well. It can also be helpful for a variety of skin issues.

Be safe: Benzoin may cause drowsiness. Benzoin may irritate sensitive skin, so do a patch test before using.

TRY IT OUT:

 Diffusion: Diffuse benzoin in the bedroom at night, to create a cozy atmosphere conducive to sleep.

 Direct inhalation: For a quick de-stressor, or a dose of emotional comfort, rub 1 drop of benzoin between your palms, place hands over your nose, and inhale deeply.

 Skincare: Create a moisturizing oil by adding 10 drops of benzoin, 6 drops of bergamot, and 4 drops of sandalwood to ¼ cup (50ml) of a carrier oil. Massage into particularly dry or chapped areas of skin for faster healing.

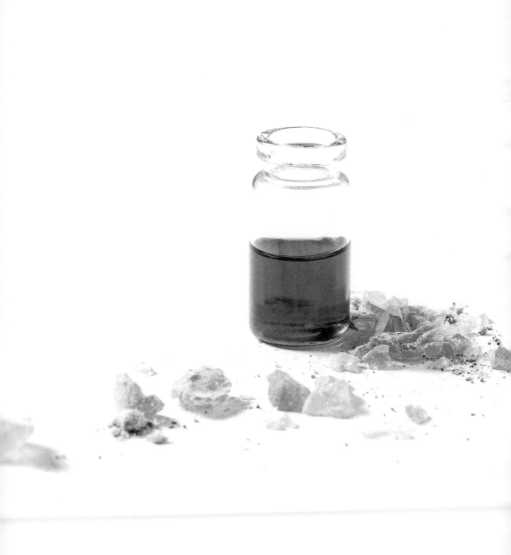

CARROT SEED

Daucus carota

 Use it for: Treating skin conditions, supporting detoxification, boosting hair health, alleviating acne, soothing muscle pain.

 Blend it with: Geranium enhances carrot seed's moisturizing properties; lemon and sweet orange boost its antiseptic and antibacterial qualities; lavender and bergamot help soothe discomfort.

What is it?: The seeds of *Daucus carota*—a wild, white-flowering herb also known as Queen Anne's lace—are dried, crushed, and steam distilled to create the earthy-smelling carrot seed essential oil. With antiseptic, antibacterial, and soothing properties, this oil is mostly known for its many skincare benefits.

Be safe: Do not use carrot seed while pregnant or breastfeeding.

TRY IT OUT:

 Massage: For a skin-nourishing massage that will also aid detoxification, add 12 drops of carrot seed, 5 drops of geranium, and 4 drops of lavender to ¼ cup (50ml) of a carrier oil. Blend and massage directly into skin.

 Skincare: To create a moisturizing face oil, add 5 drops of carrot seed, 2 drops of frankincense, and 3 drops of lavender to 2 tablespoons (30ml) of a carrier oil and blend. At night, rub 1 to 2 drops in your palms and pat over a clean face. Store in a small dark blue or amber bottle.

 Direct application: Carrot seed can have a calming effect on skin conditions such as eczema, rashes, and psoriasis. To treat, mix a couple of drops of carrot seed with a couple of drops of a carrier oil, then apply to the affected area with your fingers.

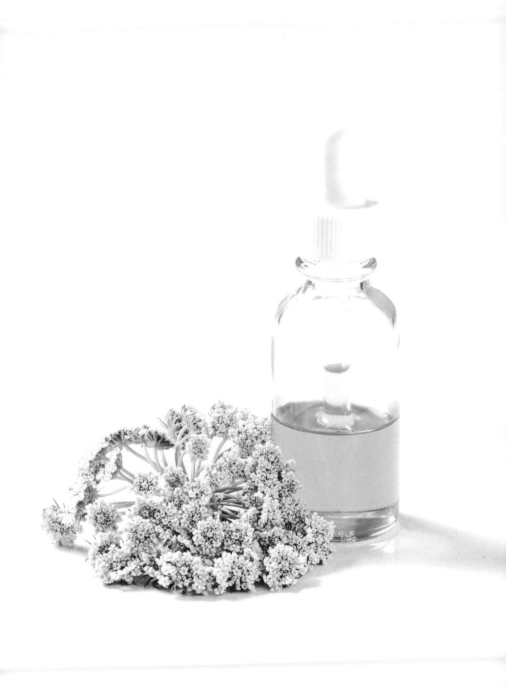

CEDARWOOD (ATLAS)

Cedrus atlantica

 Use it for: Treating an itchy, oily scalp; boosting skin and hair health; repelling insects; detoxifying; grounding emotions.

 Blend it with: Grapefruit and lemongrass help support detoxification; citronella and clove are also insect deterrents; bergamot enhances feelings of well-being.

What is it?: The tall, coniferous *Cedrus atlantica* tree, an evergreen native to North Africa, imparts its earthy, woody smell through wood chips and shavings that are steam distilled to create atlas cedarwood essential oil. Long used as an intoxicating fragrance, atlas cedarwood also has benefits for skin and hair and offers emotional support as well.

Be safe: Atlas cedarwood may irritate sensitive skin, so do a patch test before using. Do not use atlas cedarwood while pregnant or breastfeeding.

TRY IT OUT:

 Diffusion: To keep the insects at bay on warm summer nights, diffuse atlas cedarwood. Add citronella or clove to make an insect-repelling blend.

 Hair care: To treat dandruff or an itchy scalp, add a couple of drops of atlas cedarwood to 1 teaspoon of jojoba oil and massage into your scalp after shampooing, working it through to the ends of your hair.

 Indirect inhalation: For easy-to-access calming and grounding, create an aromatic spritzer. Add 10 drops of atlas cedarwood, 8 drops of bergamot, and 6 drops of ylang-ylang to ¼ cup (50ml) water in a small, portable amber or dark blue spray bottle and shake to blend. To use, spray in the air and walk through it, inhaling deeply.

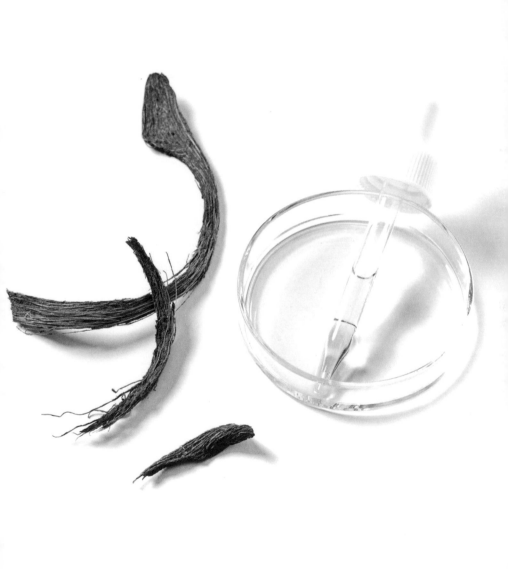

CYPRESS

Cupressus sempervirens

 Use it for: Enhancing mental clarity, boosting emotional comfort, supporting detoxification, reducing swelling, soothing inflammation.

 Blend it with: Fennel and grapefruit help with detoxification; lavender enhances its anti-inflammatory effects; the slightly sweet, fruity scent of bergamot pairs well with cypress's arboreal aroma; tea tree boosts its antibacterial nature.

What is it?: *Cupressus sempervirens* is a coniferous evergreen tree, also known as a Mediterranean cypress. Twigs and needles are steam distilled to create the clean, woody-scented cypress essential oil. This essence is used not only for its pleasing fragrance but also for its anti-inflammatory and de-stressing qualities.

Be safe: Do not use cypress while pregnant or breastfeeding.

TRY IT OUT:

 Compress: To treat joint inflammation or the swelling of an injury, create a cold compress by mixing 5 drops of cypress and 3 drops of lavender in 1 cup (250ml) iced water. Take a clean, folded facecloth and place it on top of the water, letting it soak up as much oil and water as possible. Wring out the water and place the compress on the swollen area.

 Bath: For a detoxifying bath that will also lift your mood, add 3 to 6 drops of cypress to a tablespoon of a carrier oil and add to a warm bath.

 Diffusion: Use cypress in the home, especially during the winter months, for a subtle scent that both soothes and energizes.

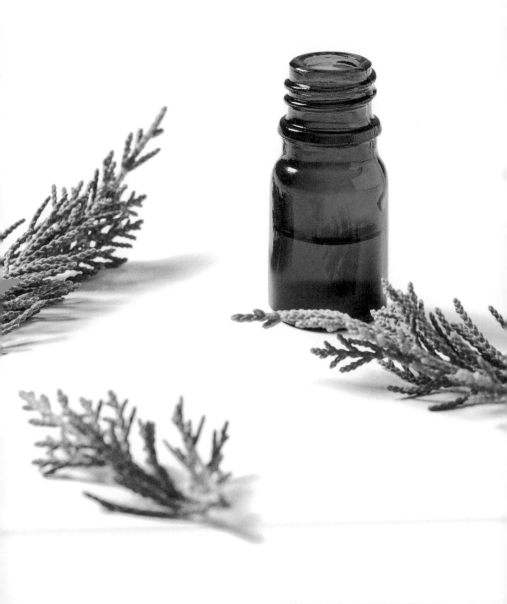

ELEMI

Canarium luzonicum

 Use it for: Calming nerves, soothing sore muscles, treating cuts and scrapes, boosting skin health.

 Blend it with: Frankincense and myrrh have similar wound-healing properties; lavender gives elemi's spiciness a floral note while boosting its relaxing effects; thyme's antibacterial properties complement elemi's skin benefits.

What is it?: Elemi essential oil is distilled from the resin of *Canarium luzonicum*, also known as the canary tree, native to the Philippines. Its scent is both citrusy and peppery, and the oil is healing for the skin, soothing for the body, and calming for the mind.

Be safe: Elemi may irritate sensitive skin, so do a patch test before using.

TRY IT OUT:

 Diffusion: Diffuse elemi with lavender in the home to create a comforting, calming environment.

 Massage: For a massage that eases muscle stiffness while nourishing skin, mix 6 drops of elemi and 4 drops of frankincense in 2 tablespoons (30ml) of a carrier oil (scale up as needed). Blend and massage directly into skin.

 Skincare: Elemi can help renew sun-damaged or lackluster skin. Add a drop to a single-use amount of your nightly moisturizer before applying.

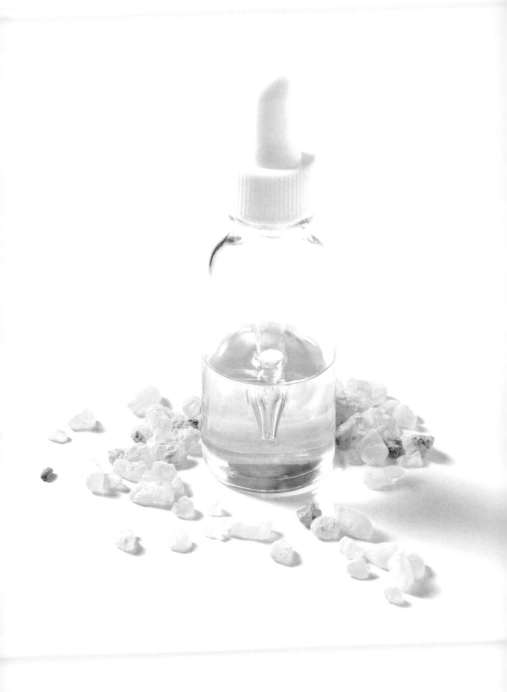

FIR NEEDLE

Abies balsamea

 Use it for: Freshening the air, cleaning the home, soothing sore muscles, boosting energy, preventing infections.

 Blend it with: Lemon and rosemary enhance its antibacterial properties; pine adds complexity to fir needle's green scent; sweet orange gives its stimulating aroma an emotional uplift.

What is it?: The needles of the *Abies balsamea*, a tall, coniferous tree, are steam distilled to create fir needle essential oil. This oil has the green, earthy scent of a freshly cut forest tree, and its analgesic and antimicrobial properties make it useful in treating the body and freshening up the home.

Be safe: Fir needle may irritate sensitive skin, so do a patch test before using.

TRY IT OUT:

 Diffusion: For a fresh, uplifting scent, diffuse fir needle with sweet orange in the home, especially if you live in an urban environment.

 Massage: To ease sore muscles, create a massage oil. Add 10 drops of fir needle to 2 tablespoons (30ml) of a carrier oil (scale up as needed). Blend and massage directly into skin.

 Home: To get the air cleaning and aromatherapeutic benefits of fir needle oil, create this room spray: mix 5 drops of fir needle, 2 drops of lemon, and 1 drop of rosemary in ¼ cup (50ml) water. Shake before using and spray as needed.

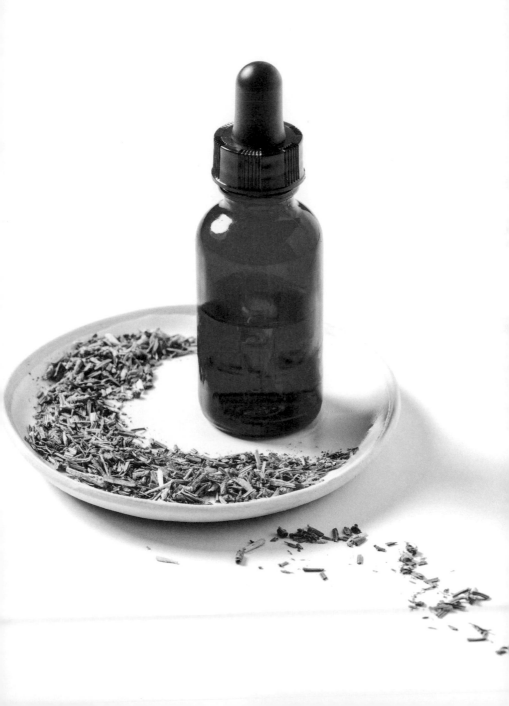

FRANKINCENSE

Boswellia carterii

 Use it for: Boosting skin health, treating cuts and scrapes, increasing energy and sense of well-being, alleviating headaches, soothing respiratory issues.

 Blend it with: Cypress and geranium also help smooth skin; lavender enhances frankincense's relaxing effects; grapefruit boosts its antiseptic properties.

What is it?: The resin of *Boswellia carterii*—a short, branchy tree topped with the stems of small green leaves—is steam distilled to make the bright, woody-spicy frankincense. Used for thousands of years as an incense and fragrance, frankincense also has many other uses, both physical (it's antiseptic and antibacterial) and emotional (it's a renowned mood booster).

Be safe: Do not use frankincense while pregnant or breastfeeding.

TRY IT OUT:

 Diffusion: Frankincense is a wonderful mood enhancer, alleviating anxiety and creating a sense of calm, while also helping with fatigue. Diffuse frankincense in the home, to create a healing environment.

 Direct inhalation: To help quickly dispel anxiety, or feelings of being overwhelmed, rub 1 drop of frankincense between your palms, place hands over your nose, and inhale deeply.

 Skincare: To give your skin a moisturizing boost, add 1 drop of frankincense to a single-use amount of your nightly moisturizer before applying to your face.

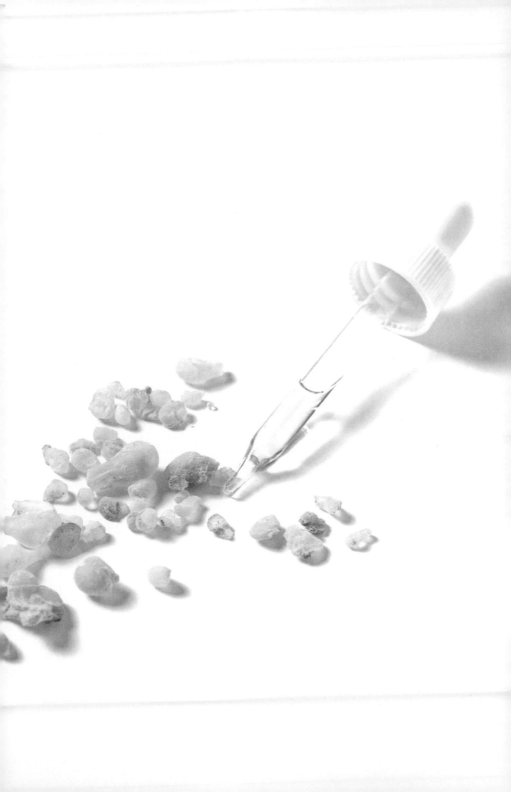

JUNIPER BERRY

Juniperus communis

 Use it for: Treating cuts and scrapes, alleviating skin issues, easing restlessness, relieving sore muscles, boosting mindfulness.

 Blend it with: Geranium helps soothe skin; clary sage and atlas cedarwood enhance juniper berry's ability to mitigate anxiety; sweet orange is also antiseptic and its citrus scent complements juniper berry's green aroma; peppermint gives it an added mental boost.

What is it?: The evergreen *Juniperus communis* can be grown as a tall tree or low shrub, with short needles and dark blue berries, which are distilled to make juniper berry essential oil.

The slightly sweet, woody aroma is subtle and fresh, and the oil is both antiseptic and analgesic in addition to having a potent emotionally grounding effect.

Be safe: Do not use juniper berry while pregnant or breastfeeding. People with kidney or liver ailments should refrain from using it.

TRY IT OUT:

 Direct application: To speed the healing of a cut, scrape, burn, or bite, mix a couple of drops of juniper berry with a few drops of a carrier oil and apply to the affected area after cleaning.

 Bath: For a skin-nourishing and mentally soothing bath, add 5 drops of juniper berry and 3 drops of geranium to a tablespoon of a carrier oil and add to a warm bath.

 Direct inhalation: For a fast and easy way to ground yourself during a stressful day, rub 1 drop of juniper berry between your palms, place hands over your nose, and inhale deeply.

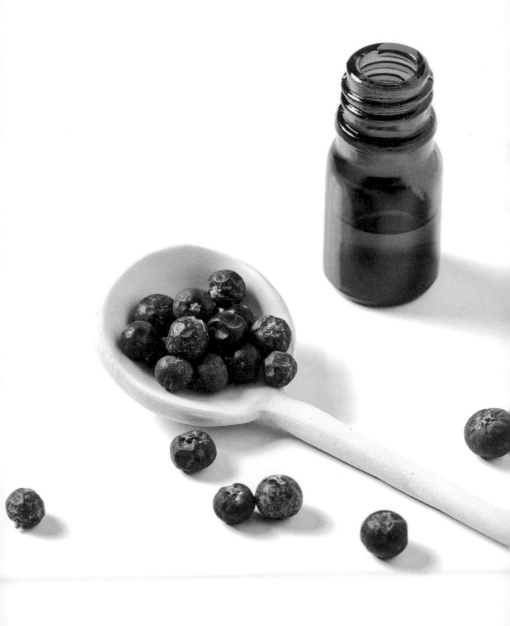

MYRRH

Commiphora myrrha

 Use it for: Brightening skin, treating small cuts and sores, alleviating skin issues and infections, boosting mouth health, calming nerves.

 Blend it with: Cypress and geranium boost its skin benefits; lavender and Roman chamomile enhance its soothing properties; clove is also good for mouth health.

What is it?: Resin from *Commiphora myrrha*, a thorny tree native to parts of the Arabian Peninsula along the Red Sea, is steam distilled to make myrrh essential oil. Its warm, spicy scent has long been used for incense and religious purposes, and it has benefits beyond aromatherapy, including its enhancement of skin and mouth health.

Be safe: Do not use myrrh internally. Do not use myrrh while pregnant or breastfeeding.

TRY IT OUT:

 Diffusion: Honor myrrh's ancient spiritual history by diffusing it during special occasions to create a peaceful, mindful environment. Add frankincense and sandalwood for a comforting, complex aroma.

 Mouth care: Myrrh's antibacterial and anti-inflammatory properties can help treat many mouth-related issues, from ulcers to gingivitis. To create a mouth rinse, mix 2 drops of myrrh in 2 tablespoons (30ml) water and swish in your mouth for 30 seconds. Do not swallow.

 Skincare: To brighten and smooth skin, create a serum. In a small amber or dark blue glass bottle with a dropper cap, mix 1 tablespoon of coconut oil, ½ tablespoon each of jojoba and aloe vera, and ½ teaspoon of vitamin E with 5 drops of myrrh, 3 drops of lavender, and 2 drops of geranium. Rub 2 drops between your palms and pat on your face in the evening after cleansing.

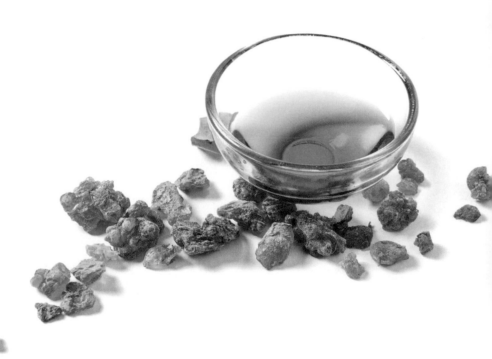

PATCHOULI

Pogostemon cablin

 Use it for: Alleviating dry skin and dandruff, repelling insects, easing stress, enhancing arousal, supporting mindfulness.

 Blend it with: The spicy scent of clove adds depth to patchouli's aroma; geranium enhances its positive effect on emotions; lemongrass helps support mindfulness; lavender and Roman chamomile boost its ability to promote relaxation.

What is it?: The leaves of *Pogostemon cablin*, a bushy flowering herb in the mint family, are steam distilled to create patchouli essential oil. The intoxicating sweet and spicy scent of patchouli has long made it a favorite for perfumes and fragrances, but its calming and astringent qualities make it great for skincare and general uplift as well.

Be safe: There are no known precautions associated with patchouli oil.

TRY IT OUT:

 Bath: For a bathing experience that will soothe your skin as well as your spirit, add 6 drops of patchouli to a tablespoon of a carrier oil and add it to a warm bath.

 Fragrance: For a sweet rich scent that can inspire calm throughout the day, place 1 drop of patchouli on the inside of each wrist.

 Skincare: To take advantage of patchouli's moisturizing and anti-inflammatory properties, mix 1 drop into your nightly face cream before applying.

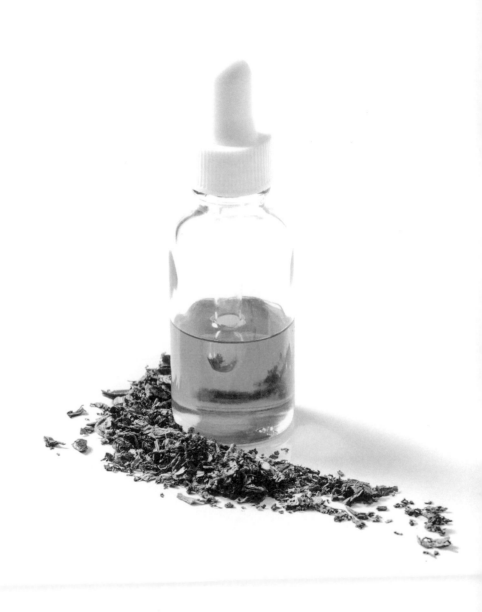

PINE

Pinus sylvestris

 Use it for: Soothing muscle pain, alleviating congestion, clearing and soothing the mind, boosting air quality, creating a seasonal winter aroma.

 Blend it with: Atlas cedarwood and eucalyptus aid its use as a decongestant; lavender complements pine's soothing elements; spruce and fir needle make it a woody powerhouse.

What is it?: Needles from the *Pinus sylvestris*—a tall, pine-coned tree—are steam distilled to create pine essential oil. Its well-known fresh scent is like having a forest in a bottle.

Pine essential oil is antiviral, antiseptic, and anti-inflammatory, making it great for treating cold and flu symptoms as well as sore and tired muscles.

Be safe: Pine may irritate sensitive skin, so do a patch test before using. Refrain from using pine if you have respiratory issues.

TRY IT OUT:

 Diffusion: Diffuse pine to increase the air quality of an environment; during the winter months, it creates a festive, soothing scent.

 Massage: To spot-treat sore muscles or joint pain, mix 10 drops of pine with 10 drops of a carrier oil (scale up as needed). Blend and massage directly into skin.

 Steam inhalation: To help clear sinuses and ease chest congestion, add 3 to 5 drops of pine to a bowl of hot water. Place a towel over your head, lean over the bowl, and inhale deeply for a minute or two.

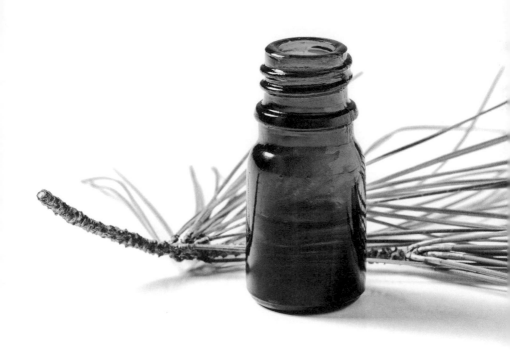

SANDALWOOD

Santalum spicatum

 Use it for: Enhancing meditation, easing anxiety, nourishing hair, boosting libido, fighting infections.

 Blend it with: Clary sage boosts sandalwood's grounding element; lemon enhances its antiseptic properties; frankincense and tangerine complement its effects on well-being; palmarosa is beneficial for hair.

What is it?: The hard, inner heartwood of *Santalum spicatum*—a small flowering tree native to Australia—is chipped and distilled to create Australian sandalwood essential oil. Though its rich, woody aroma is not quite as intense as the widely used Indian sandalwood (*Santalum album*), it has very similar properties and is a much more sustainable option. Sandalwood has been a fragrant mainstay for centuries, and it has potent emotional benefits as well as physically nourishing properties.

Be safe: Sandalwood may cause drowsiness.

TRY IT OUT:

 Direct inhalation: Use sandalwood to ground yourself and create a supportive space for meditation; rub 1 drop of the sandlewood between your palms, place hands over your nose, and inhale deeply.

 Diffusion: Take advantage of sandalwood's sensual, aphrodisiac effect by diffusing it in the bedroom.

 Hair care: For dry or brittle hair, create a hair mask with sandalwood. Add 6 drops of sandalwood, 4 drops of palmarosa, and 2 drops of lavender to 2 tablespoons (30ml) of jojoba oil. Massage into dry or damp hair from scalp to ends. Cover with a warm towel for 20 minutes to an hour, then wash as usual.

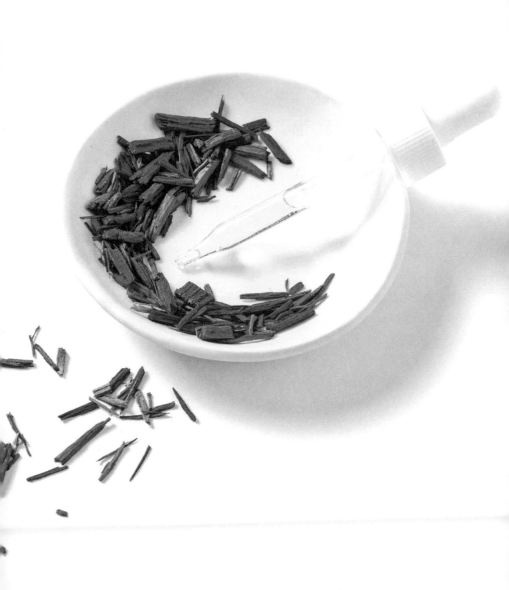

SPIKENARD

Nardostachys jatamansi

 Use it for: Easing restlessness, encouraging sleep, soothing muscle spasms, calming anxiety, boosting skin health.

 Blend it with: Roman chamomile and neroli are also helpful relaxants; petitgrain boosts spikenard's muscle-soothing properties; myrrh and rose complement its skincare benefits.

What is it?: It is the roots of *Nardostachys jatamansi*, a plant topped with clusters of tiny flowers in shades of pink, purple, and white, that are steam distilled to create the sweetly pungent spikenard oil. Spikenard has been used for centuries, and is best known for its calming and de-stressing qualities.

Be safe: Spikenard may cause drowsiness.

TRY IT OUT:

 Diffusion: For a relaxing blend to ease you into a good night's sleep, diffuse spikenard with lavender and Roman chamomile in the home, particularly the bedroom.

 Direct application: To treat anxiety and feelings of being overwhelmed, mix 1 drop of spikenard with a couple of drops of a carrier oil and apply a dab to each temple. Close your eyes, and inhale deeply and slowly.

 Skincare: Help soften skin by including spikenard in your beauty routine: add 1 drop to a single-use amount of your nightly moisturizer before applying to your face.

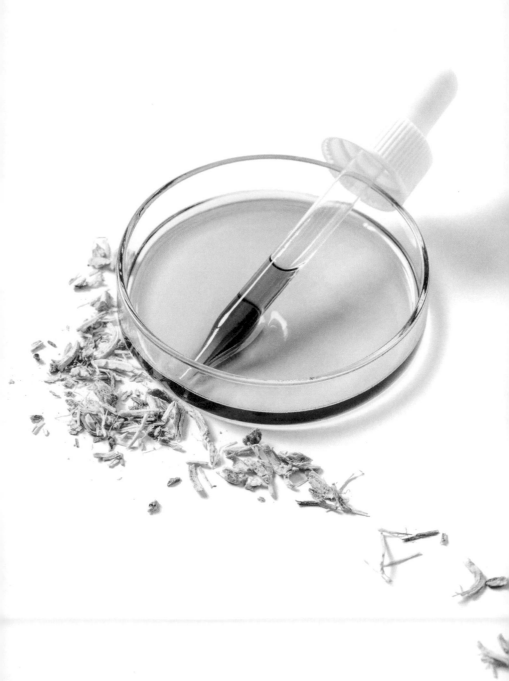

SPRUCE

Picea mariana

 Use it for: Soothing stiff muscles, treating joint pain, relieving congestion, freshening the air, easing fatigue.

 Blend it with: Blue chamomile and lavender add a calming effect; pine and rosemary can help clean the air; peppermint boosts its effect as a decongestant.

What is it?: The needles of the coniferous evergreen tree *Picea mariana* are steam distilled to create spruce essential oil. The fresh green scent of this essential oil is like bottling the aroma of a freshly felled tree. It has a range of antiseptic, anti-inflammatory, and decongestive qualities.

Be safe: Spruce may irritate sensitive skin, so do a patch test before using. Do not use spruce while pregnant or breastfeeding.

TRY IT OUT:

 Diffusion: To create a fresh, calm, uplifting environment, diffuse spruce with rosemary and lavender in the home.

 Steam inhalation: To treat the symptoms of a head cold, add 3 to 5 drops of spruce to a bowl of hot water. Place a towel over your head, lean over the bowl, and inhale deeply for a minute or two.

 Direct application: To treat the symptoms of a chest cold, try this rub: In a double boiler, melt 2 tablespoons of coconut oil with 2 tablespoons of shea butter. Remove from the heat for several minutes before mixing in 8 drops of spruce, 8 drops of peppermint, and 4 drops of lavender. Pour the blend into a glass jar with a lid and cool completely. To use, rub a small amount between your fingers and apply directly to the chest.

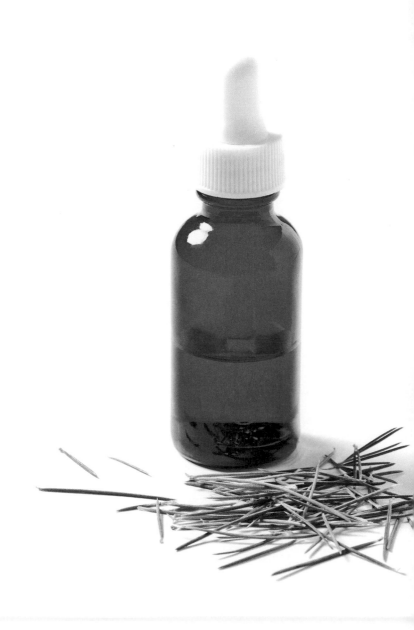

VALERIAN

Valeriana officinalis

 Use it for: Promoting sleep, easing anxiety, alleviating depression, mitigating restlessness, treating stress-related headaches.

 Blend it with: Lavender and Roman chamomile boost valerian's sleep support; mandarin and pine complement with emotional uplift; petitgrain helps with muscle-calming benefits.

What is it?: The rope-like roots of *Valeriana officinalis*, a tall, bushy herb topped with clusters of small pink or white flowers, are steam distilled to create valerian essential oil. Long used in homeopathy because of its sedative properties, this funky, medicinal-smelling oil is helpful for all manner of emotional, mental, and physical calming.

Be safe: Valerian may irritate sensitive skin, so do a patch test before using. Valerian may cause drowsiness. Do not use valerian while pregnant or breastfeeding.

TRY IT OUT:

 Bath: For a calming bath that will also improve your sense of well-being, add 3 drops of valerian and 4 drops of mandarin to a tablespoon of a carrier oil and add it to a warm bath.

 Diffusion: Diffuse valerian with lavender and Roman chamomile in the bedroom at night to help combat insomnia and restless leg syndrome.

 Massage: Use valerian in a massage oil to amplify its relaxing effects. Add 4 drops of valerian, 3 drops of petitgrain, and 5 drops of lavender to 2 tablespoons (30ml) of a carrier oil (scale up as needed). Blend and massage directly into skin.

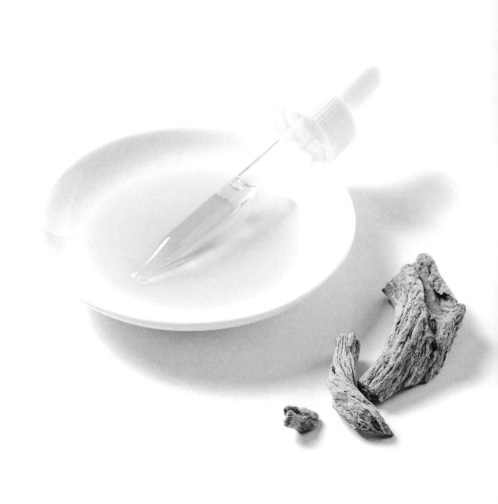

VETIVER

Vetiveria zizanoides

 Use it for: Increasing concentration, easing restlessness, uplifting emotions, soothing muscle and joint pain.

 Blend it with: Bergamot and clary sage enhance vetiver's uplifting effects while boosting its grounding properties; lavender and spikenard are also powerful relaxants; jasmine aids in concentration.

What is it?: The dried roots of *Vetiveria zizanoides*, a tall, skinny grass, are distilled to create vetiver essential oil. It has a strong woody, earthy scent and is a popular (and powerful!) base note in fragrances. It's emotionally beneficial and has analgesic, anti-inflammatory, and antiseptic properties as well.

Be safe: Vetiver may cause drowsiness.

TRY IT OUT:

 Bath: If you're feeling overwhelmed or irritable, try taking a bath with vetiver. Add 3 drops of vetiver to a tablespoon of a carrier oil and add to a warm bath.

 Diffusion: Vetiver is great for diffusion, but it's best blended with other oils to dilute its viscosity. Diffuse with bergamot and clary sage for overall well-being and with lavender for an especially relaxing experience.

 Direct application: Treat sunburned skin with vetiver's cooling, soothing properties. In a small spray bottle, add 6 drops of vetiver and 4 drops of lavender to ¼ cup (50ml) of aloe vera juice. Shake to blend before spraying onto the affected area.

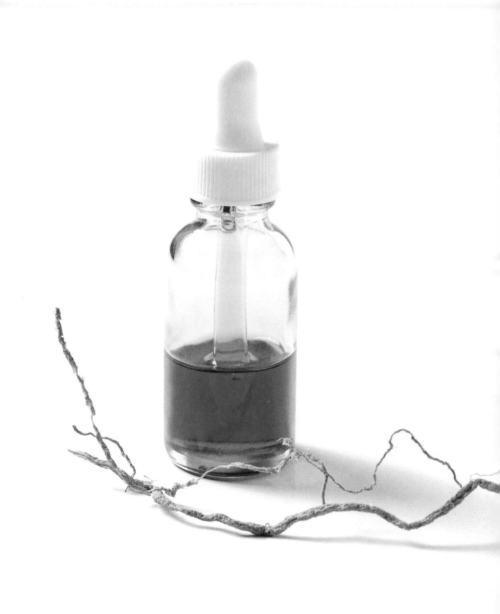

BERGAMOT

Citrus bergamia

 Use it for: Soothing inflammation, de-stressing, emotional uplift, treating infections, boosting hair health.

 Blend it with: Black pepper and niaouli provide additional immune support; mandarin boosts bergamot's citrus scent and mood-enhancing properties; rose complements its calming effects; cypress has similar anti-inflammatory benefits.

What is it?: The rinds of the fruit of *Citrus bergamia* are cold pressed to create bergamot essential oil, which has a slightly sweet and spicy citrus-floral scent. Used in fragrances for its inviting aroma, bergamot oil is also a powerful mood lifter with antibiotic, analgesic, and antiseptic properties as well.

Be safe: Bergamot is a photosensitizer; do not use on skin that may be exposed to the sun.

TRY IT OUT:

 Bath: For a stress-relieving, immunity-boosting bath, add 5 drops of bergamot and 2 drops of niaouli to a tablespoon of a carrier oil and add to a warm bath.

 Diffusion: Diffuse bergamot in the home to raise spirits, promote sleep, and create an aromatic blend with a wide range of other oils.

 Direct inhalation: For a quick and easy way to elevate your mood, rub 1 drop of bergamot between your palms, place hands over your nose, and inhale deeply.

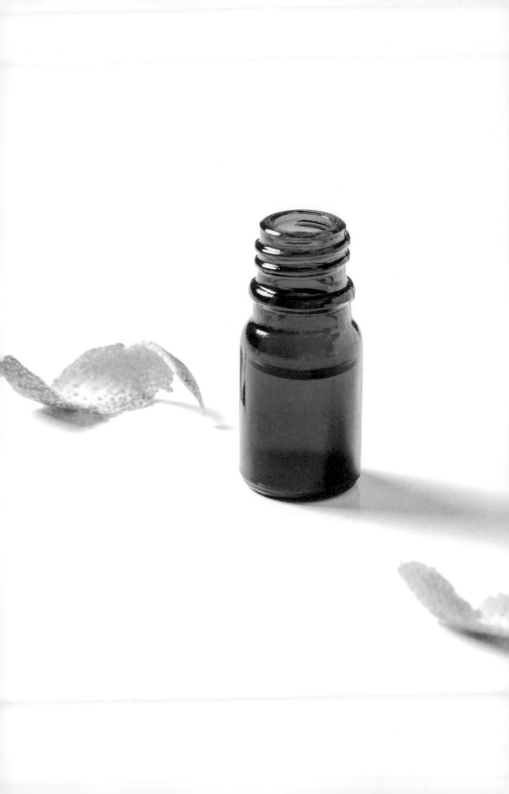

CITRONELLA

Cymbopogon nardus

 Use it for: Repelling insects, soothing joint pain, freshening the air, alleviating foot odor, mitigating fatigue.

 Blend it with: Atlas cedarwood and lemongrass boost its insect-repelling properties; sweet orange enhances its energizing effects; the floral scent of lavender and spicy-citrus aroma of bergamot complement citronella's air-freshening abilities.

What is it?: *Cymbopogon nardus*, a tall, bushy grass native to tropical regions of Asia, is steam distilled to create citronella essential oil. The earthy, citrusy oil has anti-inflammatory and antibacterial properties, and though it's most well known as an insect repellent, it has many other uses as well.

Be safe: Citronella may irritate sensitive skin, so do a patch test before using. Do not use citronella while pregnant or breastfeeding.

TRY IT OUT:

 Diffusion: Diffuse citronella in the home, especially near openings, such as windows and doors, to deter insects.

 Home: For an easy bathroom air freshener, mix the following in a small spray bottle: ¼ cup (50ml) water, 5 drops of citronella, 5 drops of lavender, and 2 drops of bergamot. Shake to blend and spray as needed.

 Massage: For stiff muscles or inflamed joints, create a massage oil. Add 10 drops of citronella to 2 tablespoons (30ml) of a carrier oil (scale up as needed). Blend and massage directly into skin.

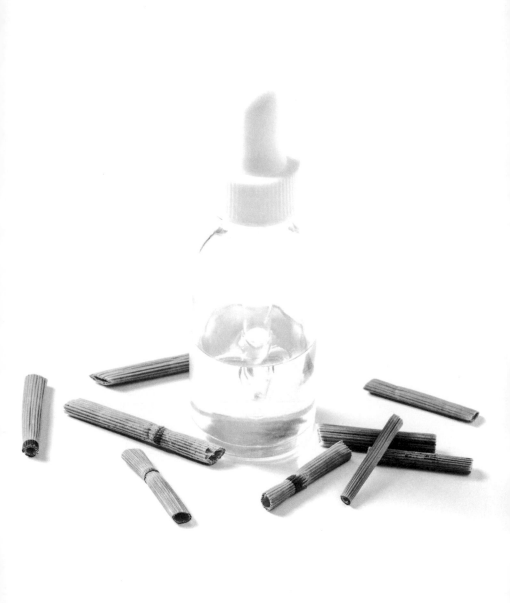

GRAPEFRUIT

Citrus paradisi

 Use it for: Easing the symptoms of motion sickness, supporting detoxification, enhancing a sense of well-being, treating oily skin and scalp, curbing sugar cravings.

 Blend it with: Sweet orange has similar antibacterial benefits; juniper is good for oily skin while rosemary helps treat an oily scalp; peppermint boosts its craving-curbing properties; ylang-ylang's floral fragrance pairs well with grapefruit's citrus scent and alleviates feelings of depression.

What is it?: Rinds from the fruit of the *Citrus paradisi* tree are cold pressed to create sweetly refreshing grapefruit essential oil. Like other citrus essences, grapefruit is uplifting and energizing as well as being antiseptic and beneficial to the skin and hair.

Be safe: Grapefruit may irritate sensitive skin, so do a patch test before using. Grapefruit oil is a photosensitizer; do not use on skin that may be exposed to the sun.

TRY IT OUT:

 Bath: For a detoxifying bath that will also lift your spirits, add 5 drops of grapefruit and 3 drops of ylang-ylang to a tablespoon of a carrier oil and add to a warm bath.

 Direct inhalation: To calm feelings of nausea or dissipate the need for a sweet treat, rub 1 drop of grapefruit between your palms, place hands over your nose, and inhale deeply.

 Skincare: Grapefruit has astringent qualities that make it useful for treating oily skin. To make a toner, add 6 drops of grapefruit to 2 tablespoons (30ml) of witch hazel in a small amber or dark blue bottle. To use, shake to blend, dab onto a cotton ball, and wipe over your face after cleansing.

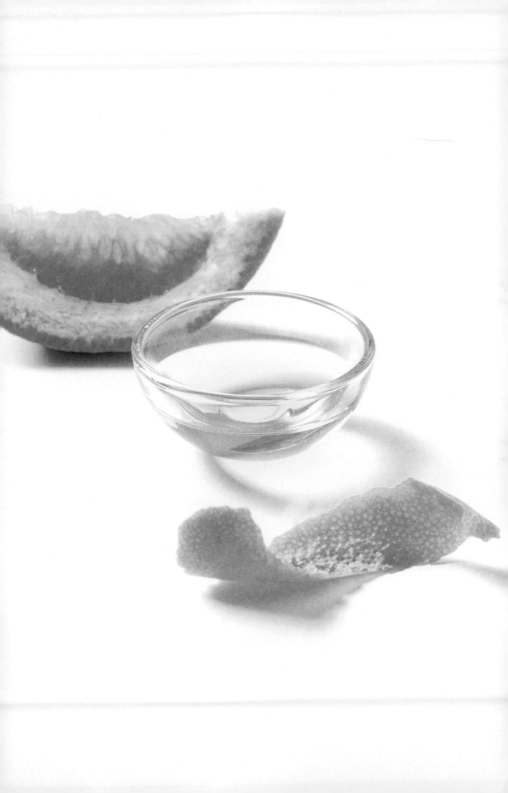

LEMON

Citrus limon

 Use it for: Boosting the immune system, reinvigorating the mind, alleviating a cough or sore throat, soothing a headache, cleaning the house.

 Blend it with: Lavender and peppermint help ease a cough/sore throat; sweet orange and eucalyptus boost its antiseptic properties; tangerine complements its invigorating scent.

What is it?: Fresh rinds from the fruit of the *Citrus limon* tree are cold pressed to create this bright citrus oil. This well-known scent is very therapeutic, and because of the essential oil's antimicrobial properties, it's also great for household cleaning.

Be safe: Lemon may irritate sensitive skin, so do a patch test before using. Cold-pressed lemon oil is a photosensitizer; do not use on skin that may be exposed to the sun.

TRY IT OUT:

 Direct inhalation: To alleviate the symptoms of a headache, rub a drop of lemon oil between your palms, place hands over your nose, and inhale deeply.

 Home: To make an all-purpose soft scrub cleanser, combine ¼ cup (50ml) of castile soap, ¾ cup (180g) of baking soda, 10 drops of lemon, and 10 drops of sweet orange in a jar. To use, apply to surfaces with a damp cloth.

 Mouth care: To ease a sore throat, mix 5 drops of lemon and 1 tablespoon of honey in a cup of warm water. Gargle for 15 seconds and spit it out. Repeat until the cup is empty.

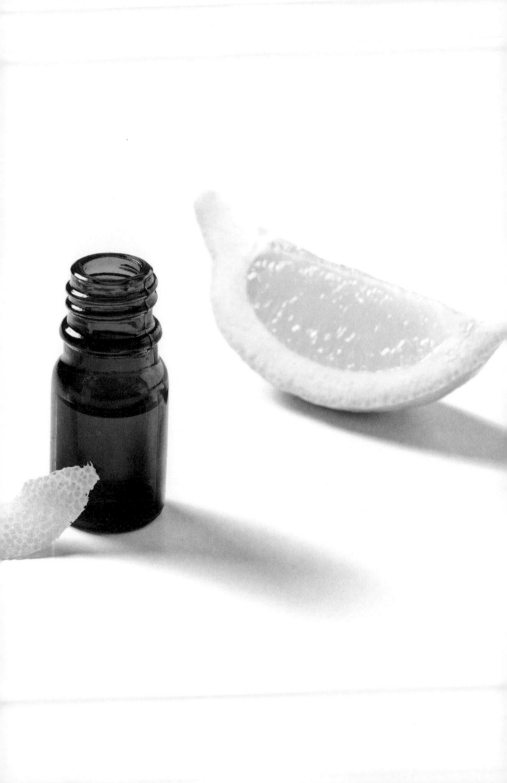

LIME

Citrus aurantifolia

 Use it for: Alleviating the blues, enhancing mental acuity, treating oily skin and scalp, boosting the immune system, cleaning the home.

 Blend it with: Bergamot and lemon amp up lime's citrus, mood-boosting scent; clary sage adds a grounding element to its uplifting properties; benzoin's vanilla aroma adds warmth to lime's brightness; lavendin is a complementary de-stressor.

What is it?: The rind from the fruits of the *Citrus aurantifolia* tree, aka lime tree, is cold pressed to create this bright, tart citrus oil. Lime is a reliable mood booster, great for an emotional and mental pick-me-up, and has many practical uses as well.

Be safe: Lime may irritate sensitive skin, so do a patch test before using. Lime oil is a photosensitizer; do not use on skin that may be exposed to the sun.

TRY IT OUT:

 Diffusion: To brighten an environment and lift your mood, especially during the dark winter months, diffuse lime in the home.

 Home: For a glass and mirror cleaner, mix 1 cup (250ml) of white vinegar with 1 cup (250ml) water in a spray bottle. Add 15 drops of lime and shake to combine.

 Hair care: To combat a sebaceous scalp, add 1 to 2 drops of lime to a single-use amount of shampoo before massaging into scalp and washing as usual.

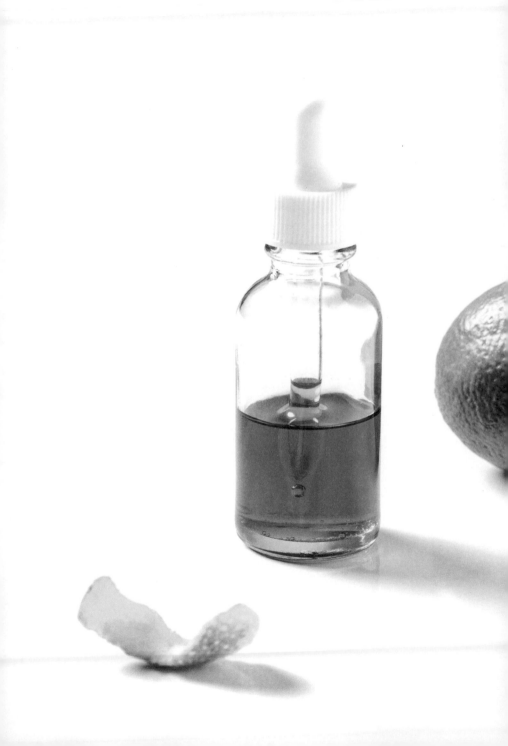

MANDARIN

Citrus reticulata

 Use it for: Supporting sleep, lifting spirits, boosting skin health, relieving indigestion, cleaning the home.

 Blend it with: Geranium and jasmine complement its skin benefits; lavender and Roman chamomile enhance mandarin's soothing effect; grapefruit boosts its citrus scent and antibacterial properties.

What is it?: The rind of the small orange fruits of the *Citrus reticulata* tree is cold pressed to create mandarin essential oil. This sweet citrus oil is uplifting and gentle, with properties that benefit the body and the home.

Be safe: Mandarin oil is a photosensitizer; do not use on skin that may be exposed to the sun.

TRY IT OUT:

 Diffusion: For a bit of sunshine during the winter months, diffuse mandarin in the home to create a cheery environment.

 Home: Freshen up the air in a room with this aromatic blend: add 5 drops of mandarin, 3 drops of grapefruit, and 2 drops of lavender to 1 cup (250ml) water in a spray bottle. Spray as needed, shaking to blend before each use.

 Skincare: To reap mandarin's skin-softening benefits, add a couple of drops to a single-use amount of your body lotion before applying directly to skin.

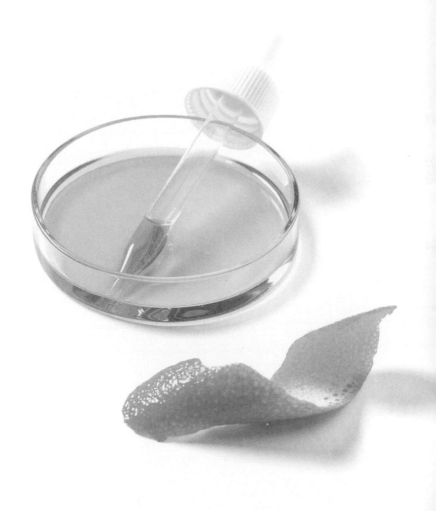

SWEET ORANGE

Citrus sinensis

 Use it for: De-stressing, mitigating anxiety, uplifting emotions, alleviating insomnia, soothing headaches.

 Blend it with: Eucalyptus and melissa complement sweet orange's mood-enhancing effects; peppermint and rosemary help treat headaches; the scent of jasmine complements its bright citrus scent.

What is it?: Fresh rinds from the fruit of the *Citrus sinensis* tree are cold pressed or distilled to create this sweet, warm citrus oil. Sweet orange is an emotionally therapeutic powerhouse and has antibacterial and detoxifying properties as well.

Be safe: Sweet orange essential oil is a photosensitizer; do not use on skin that may be exposed to the sun.

TRY IT OUT:

 Direct inhalation: For an instant mood booster, rub 1 drop of sweet orange oil between your palms, place hands over your nose, and inhale deeply.

 Diffusion: Diffuse sweet orange with clove during the winter months for a festive, uplifting scent.

 Skincare: Create a body scrub to get sweet orange's aromatic benefits while nourishing your skin as well. Add 20 drops of sweet orange to ½ cup (120ml) of jojoba oil. Mix the combined oils with 7 ounces (200g) of demerara sugar. Apply scrub directly to skin in the shower.

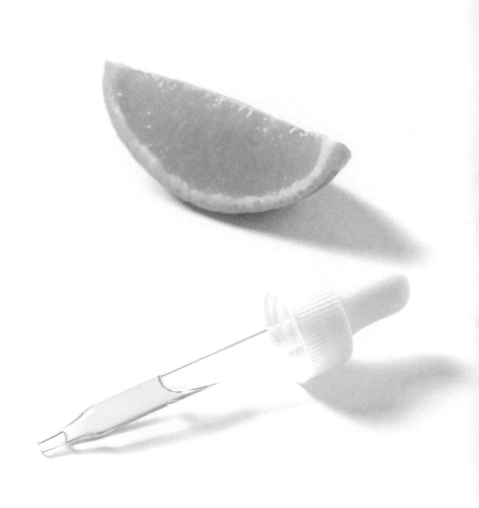

TANGERINE

Citrus reticulata

 Use it for: Boosting overall mood, reenergizing, supporting detoxification, treating digestive issues, cleaning the home.

 Blend it with: Other citrus scents, such as lemon and grapefruit, enhance its mood-boosting properties; clary sage complements its grounding effect; the floral scent of jasmine pairs well with tangerine's brightness; nutmeg is also beneficial for gastrointestinal issues.

What is it?: The rind of the small orange fruit from a tree in the *Citrus reticulata* family is cold pressed to create tangerine essential oil. It has a sweet, bright scent and wonderful emotional benefits, as well as antiseptic and antimicrobial properties that make it very useful in the home.

Be safe: Tangerine may irritate sensitive skin, so do a patch test before using. Tangerine oil is a photosensitizer; do not use on skin that may be exposed to the sun.

TRY IT OUT:

 Diffusion: Tangerine is especially good for diffusing at home during the winter months—it's like bringing a bit of sunshine inside.

 Direct inhalation: For a sweet burst of energy, rub 1 drop of tangerine between your palms, place hands over your nose, and inhale deeply.

 Shower: Add tangerine to your shower for a bright, refreshing experience that will improve your mood and boost your concentration. After washing, with the hot water still running, apply 3 drops of tangerine to a facecloth and rub it over your body, inhaling deeply as you do.

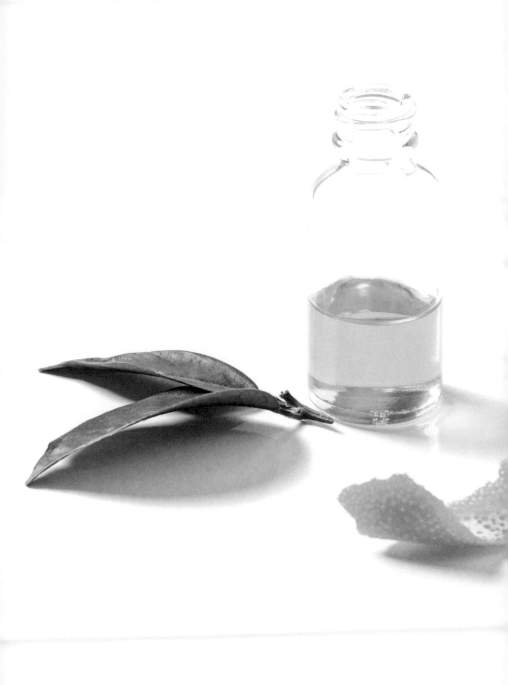

VERBENA

Lippia javanica

 Use it for: Promoting relaxation, easing anxiety, soothing muscle spasms, boosting the immune system, treating acne.

 Blend it with: Elemi enhances verbena's muscle-soothing properties; neroli helps calm the mind and body; palmarosa boosts verbena's emotionally uplifting effects; lemon adds immune boosting.

What is it?: The leaves of *Lippia javanica*, a member of the Verbenaceae family, are steam distilled to create this citrusy, herbaceous oil. It's a powerful helper when it comes to relaxing the mind and the body, and is also useful for providing an emotional boost.

Be safe: Verbena may irritate sensitive skin, so do a patch test before using. Verbena oil is a photosensitizer; do not use on skin that may be exposed to the sun.

TRY IT OUT:

 Diffusion: For an emotional uplift when you're feeling low, diffuse verbena in the home to help foster a calm, cheery environment.

 Massage: To help ease the discomfort of muscle spasms, create a massage oil. Add 6 drops of verbena, 4 drops of neroli, and 2 drops of elemi to 2 tablespoons (30ml) of a carrier oil (scale up as needed). Blend and massage directly into affected area.

 Indirect inhalation: Encourage peaceful sleep and prevent middle-of-the-night anxieties by adding a couple of drops of verbena to your pillowcase before going to bed.

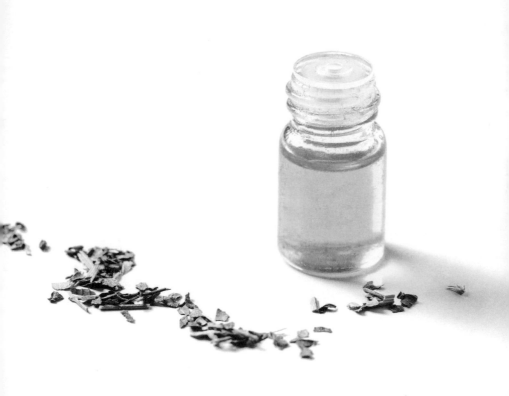

INDEX

Acknowledgments

My first thanks goes to one of my earliest yoga teachers—I no longer remember her name, but I'll never forget that she placed a drop of sweet orange oil in our palms at the end of every class, awakening me to the power of essential oils. Thanks to Catie Ziller for indulging my love of oils, to Kathy Steer for wrangling my words, and to Michelle Tilly for her gorgeous design. Thanks to dream team Julia Stotz, whose eye for beauty is unparalleled, and oil whisperer Sam Margherita. I couldn't have written a word without the gift of baby-free time from my parents and in-laws and I greatly appreciate my partner's olfactory tolerance and moral support through the process. Extra-special thanks to the plants, for the beauty, wisdom, and healing they offer.

Copyright © 2019 by Hachette Livre (Marabout)
All rights reserved.
Published in the United States by Harmony Books, an imprint of Random House, a division of Penguin Random House LLC, New York.
harmonybooks.com
Harmony Books is a registered trademark, and the Circle colophon is a trademark of Penguin Random House LLC.

Originally published in French in France as *Guide des Huiles essentielles pour debutantes* by Marabout, a member of Hachette Livre, Paris, in 2019. Copyright © 2019 by Hachette Livre (Marabout).

Library of Congress Cataloging-in-Publication Data
Names: Butterworth, Lisa, 1977- author.
Title: A beginner's guide to essential oils : 65+ essential oils for a healthy mind and body / Lisa Butterworth.
Other titles: Guide des Huiles essentielles pour debutantes. English
Description: New York : Harmony Books, [2019]
Identifiers: LCCN 2019015960| ISBN 9780593135990 (paperback) | ISBN 9780593136003 (ebook)
Subjects: LCSH: Essences and essential oils. | Aromatherapy. | BISAC: HEALTH & FITNESS / Aromatherapy. | HEALTH & FITNESS / Naturopathy. | HEALTH & FITNESS / Alternative Therapies.

Classification: LCC RM666.A68 B8813 2019 | DDC 615.3/219–dc23
ISBN 978-0-593-13599-0
Ebook ISBN 978-0-593-13600-3
Printed in China

Book design by Michelle Tilly
Cover and book photography by Julia Stotz
Cover design by Sonia Persad
10 9 8 7 6 5 4 3 2 1
First US Edition